What Seems to be the Trouble?

To Fraser, with love

What Seems to be the Trouble?

Stories in illness and healthcare

Trisha Greenhalgh

Professor of Primary Health Care
University College London

Foreword by
Sir Kenneth Calman

Vice Chancellor
Durham University

Radcliffe Publishing
Oxford • Seattle

Radcliffe Publishing Ltd
18 Marcham Road
Abingdon
Oxon OX14 1AA
United Kingdom

www.radcliffe-oxford.com
Electronic catalogue and worldwide online ordering facility.

British Library Cataloguing in Publication Data

A catalogue record for this book is available from the British Library.

ISBN-10: 1 84619 122 X
ISBN-13: 978 1 84619 122 0

Typeset by Anne Joshua & Associates, Oxford
Printed and bound by TJ International Ltd, Padstow, Cornwall

Contents

Foreword

I've always been interested in how people learn, especially doctors and other health professionals. In recently reviewing the history of medical education I have noted that the methods of learning which have been used have been relatively limited – books, lectures, tutorials, laboratory work, clinical teaching, and more recently problem-based learning and the increasing use of computers. However, throughout the long recorded history, the telling of stories has been an important part of the process. Stories are, as Professor Greenhalgh notes, 'natural and universal forms of communication'. The range of stories has extended from the case studies recorded by Hippocrates to extensive programmes of narrative, many of which are described in this book.

Learning involves the acquisition of knowledge, skills and attitudes which help to shape practice, and it raises awareness of particular patient problems. Stories, as is well illustrated in this book, are complex, multi-layered, capable of several different interpretations, and relevant to different people in different ways depending upon their backgrounds and the context of the story. Take any group of students, doctors, patients or the public and use one of Professor Greenhalgh's stories. Watch the various responses. Even better, following the discussion ask each person to tell you what they learned from the narrative, and again the responses will vary. As Professor Greenhalgh points out, those who are uncomfortable with narrative as a tool for learning or as a method of assessment seem to want a clear objective and outcome from the process – a precise, measurable end point. This is too simplistic and does not recognise the richness and sophistication of the learning experience which can be obtained through narrative.

Stories are therefore very flexible learning tools. They can be real, as narrated by a patient or family member, or delivered in the literature by an author who uses his or her experience to illuminate some part of the human condition. Poetry, plays and novels would be examples of this form of story, and they are increasingly being used in the education of health professionals.

This book covers many of the issues associated with the power of stories, and it describes the range of situations in which they can be used – in illness, healing, organisations, research and ethics. In each of these areas the methodology is carefully examined and developed, and the role of narrative in expanding the evidence base is outlined. Stories record individual events involving particular people in particular circumstances. They need to be connected to other stories and other forms of evidence in order to put them in context and allow wider lessons to be drawn. The student, patient or member of the public needs to think beyond this one story to the general conclusions, otherwise the story will merely become an anecdote that can be used without reference to the broader knowledge base, and the next patient (also an individual) with a different story (also specific to him or her) will not benefit from the learning experience. Professor Greenhalgh's views on evidence-based medicine which are described in the book reflect her wish to go beyond the technical nature of decision making based on protocols and check lists, in order to view the individual and the context of the problem in a more holistic way. Many will agree with this approach, recognising that the need to increase the knowledge base through whatever means will be valuable, and that randomised clinical trials and laboratory research have an important place in improving care.

Stories are also ways in which doctors communicate with each other. They tell each other stories about the patients they have seen, ask for advice through stories, and are able to share some of the pain and the pleasure of caring for patients in the process.

Stories can also be a means of transmitting ideas. Indeed I introduced the concept of the Transmid to illustrate this, and used an infectious disease analogy to expand its value. Here the story is used to create and describe a new idea which the listener can consider. The contagion may be active immediately and the idea may be accepted. Alternatively, to stretch the analogy further, there may be resistance, or the idea may lie dormant for some time before being revisited in the future. The story, and hence the Transmid, is the effector arm of the initiation of change (Calman, 2000).

It is a real privilege to listen to the stories of patients and their families, to hear details of personal events, comedies and tragedies, and to use the skills of listening and interpreting to make sense of the story and together with the patient to determine whether the 'broken story' can be fixed. This book presents an excellent exploration of the issues. Its analytical and methodological approach is invaluable as people re-define illness into different categories such as 'not sick', 'not yet sick', 'inexplicably sick' and 'definitely sick'. I have written elsewhere that the history of medicine is simply the re-classification of disease. Here are some new ways of classifying the issues with which we are faced in an effort to assist in the process of healing, which is the ultimate aim of the doctor and other health professionals.

Sir Kenneth Calman
April 2006

Reference

Calman KC (2000) *A Study of Story Telling, Humour and Learning in Medicine.* London: The Stationery Office.

Preface

Narrative medicine has emerged in the last few years as a new and fascinating subject in its own right. Like all new academic subjects it relates closely to others, especially to literature, drama and linguistics.

In medical practice, however, it is increasingly important, since it opens for analysis the very heart of the patient's story and can often reveal hidden meaning. This can help patients to express themselves more easily by being better understood and so help doctors to respond more sensitively.

It is no accident that the medical implications of narratives were developed by general practitioners because they, more than any other kind of doctor, have, on average, the longest lasting relationships in medicine and so hear more medical stories. Narrative medicine can be seen as a subset of the patient–doctor relationship. As John Fry, a general practitioner from Beckenham, was the longest serving Trustee in the history of The Nuffield Trust, it is an appropriate topic for his memorial lecture. Professors of General Practice/Primary Care, especially in London and Birmingham, have been in the lead in researching this, and none more so than Professor Greenhalgh.

Much of medical practice, especially in general practice and psychiatry, consists of people telling their story. Such activities have tended to be undervalued in the past, indeed often students and trainees have been trained to interrupt and force the patient's story into the format of a conventional medical history. But telling one's story is affirming, particularly for those in distress, and many people feel better just for doing so and being listened to with respect.

For doctors and nurses, especially in primary care, the power and privilege of hearing, first hand, the story and key events in many people's lives is one of the great privileges of the role and a source of unending interest.

Analysing the patient's narrative and the subsequent dialogue in detail has become a professional process. The Trustees and staff of The Nuffield Trust are most grateful to Professor Greenhalgh for illuminating this subject so skilfully.

Sir Denis Pereira Gray OBE, HonDSc, FRCGP, FMedSci
Chairman of the Trustees
April 2006

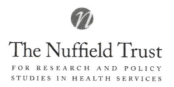

The Nuffield Trust

FOR RESEARCH AND POLICY
STUDIES IN HEALTH SERVICES

The Nuffield Trust is one of the leading independent health policy charitable trusts in the UK. It was established as the Nuffield Provincial Hospitals Trust in 1940 by Viscount Nuffield (William Morris), the founder of Morris Motors. In 1998 the Trustees agreed that the official name of the Trust should more fully reflect the Trust's purposes and, in consultation with the Charity Commission, adopted the name The Nuffield Trust for Research and Policy Studies in Health Services, retaining 'The Nuffield Trust' as its working name.

The Nuffield Trust's mission is to promote independent analysis and informed debate on UK healthcare policy. The Nuffield Trust's purpose is to communicate evidence and encourage an exchange around developed or developing knowledge in order to illuminate recognised and emerging issues.

It achieves this through its principal activities.

- Bringing together a wide national and international network of people involved in UK healthcare through a series of meetings, workshops and seminars.
- Commissioning research through its publications and grants programme to inform policy debate.
- Encouraging inter-disciplinary exchange between clinicians, legislators, academics, healthcare professionals and management, policy makers, industrialists and consumer groups.
- Supporting evidence-based health policy and practice.
- Sharing its knowledge in the home countries and internationally through partnerships and alliances.

To find out more, please refer to our website or contact:

The Nuffield Trust
59 New Cavendish St
London
W1G 7LP
Website: www.nuffieldtrust.org.uk
Email: mail@nuffieldtrust.org.uk
Tel: +44 (0)20 7631 8458
Fax: +44 (0)20 7631 8451

Charity number: 209201

About the author

Trisha Greenhalgh is a part time GP in north London and Professor of Primary Health Care at University College London. She graduated from Clare College, Cambridge in Social and Political Sciences in 1980, and gained her medical degree from University College Oxford in 1983. She began her research career at the Whittington Hospital, London in 1986, looking at the effects of emotional stress on the kinetics of insulin absorption in diabetes. Her research interests soon moved beyond the laboratory to the illness narratives and life stories of people with chronic conditions, and more recently to the organisation and delivery of health services, to which she has applied a narrative approach. She has developed a number of research, teaching and professional development programmes around these themes. Her work has a particular focus on diabetes and other chronic conditions in minority ethnic groups and the socially excluded. She was awarded the OBE for Services to Medicine in 2001.

Acknowledgements

I am indebted to many people, too numerous to mention individually, for the many influences over the years that led both directly and indirectly to this monograph. Thanks are especially due to:

- my patients, for their stories and trust
- my colleagues, for their expectations and guidance
- my students, for their questions and doubts
- my family, for their love and encouragement
- The Nuffield Trust, for an opportunity.

The following people read earlier drafts of this monograph and provided invaluable feedback: Karyn Baum, Sir Denis Pereira Gray, Andrew Herxheimer, Fraser Macfarlane, Marshall Marinker and Jill Russell. Responsibility for errors is mine alone.

Trisha Greenhalgh
April 2006

'We are never more (and sometimes less) than the co-authors of our own narratives. . . . We enter upon a stage which we did not design and we find ourselves part of an action that was not of our making. Each of us being a main character in his own drama plays subordinate parts in the dramas of others, and each drama constrains the others.'

Alasdair MacIntyre, *After Virtue*

Chapter One

Stories and illness

Vikram was born in June, June of 2002. Normal delivery, normal, no problems. That was in June, the last week of June. And around the mid-July, it was when we for the first time we felt that he wasn't feeding very well. Now, when we say he wasn't feeding very well, he used to take an awful long time to drink maybe 30 or 50 ml of normal milk, of SMA milk. He was on his mother's milk as well, but he wasn't doing very well on his mother's milk either. He was taking a really long while to drink. We mentioned this to the health visitor and she said 'that's okay, that's something, some babies do take long'. We also didn't give it too much attention because [son's name], that's his older brother, he was a fussy eater, he was a fussy drinker and he still is. So we thought, possibly Vikram is also like that.

But eventually it did become a problem in that he didn't get enough milk with that, in that he wasn't taking enough. We went to the GP a few times but nothing really happened. And then we also realised that he was coughing more than normal. And it wasn't a normal cough. So we mentioned this again, again they said it was something common, go away. And one other thing that we noticed at that time was that the back of his head when he was sleeping was getting all wet. Wet with sweat and his pillow was getting all wet, soggy. So we again mentioned this to the GP when we went and he said that was something that would go away. But nothing really happened.

Then on the 23 September, that was the day he was actually diagnosed, and on that day, that morning really we noticed he was coughing very bad. And this cough was much different than the cough that he'd had all along. And it was quite bad and it was not a normal cough, really bad. So we took him to the GP and we said 'please listen to what is, see what his problem is', and then the GP said 'I hear a murmur in his heart, can you go to the hospital?' And they wanted us to go to the hospital. We went there and we were there all day and towards the end of the day they said that they suspected a hole in the heart which is the VSD [ventricular septal defect].

Vikram's father, Database of Individual Patient Experience
www.dipex.org.uk

In one of the great works of literary analysis, *Poetics*, Aristotle proposed that a story (narrative)[1] has a number of defining characteristics, including chronology (the unfolding of events and actions over time), characters (people of greater or lesser virtue who take action and/or respond to the actions of others), context (the local and wider world in which the characters enact their business), emplotment (the rhetorical juxtaposition of events and actions to evoke meaning, motive and causality), and trouble (*peripeteia* – a breach from the expected, as in surprise or 'twist in the plot') (Aristotle, 1996b).

Chronology – the time dimension of narrative – is not merely the date-stamping of events. Philosopher Paul Ricoeur has been keen to emphasise the difference between cosmic time (measured by clocks, calendars and, ultimately, the movement of the planetary bodies) and 'event time' (measured by the significant happenings in a personal story as the narrator chooses to tell it). An interpreter told of a consultation with the refugee mother of a 16-year-old African boy with suspected psychosis. The psychiatrist asked 'How long has he been behaving like this?', to which the reply came 'Since he saw me gang-raped'. The mother's response, given in event time, provided infinitely more useful information about the boy's illness than a response expressed in cosmic time. Indeed, for Ricoeur, the chronology of narrative emerges from the interface between cosmic time (which has common significance for all of us) and event time (which is particular to each of us) – as in 'Vikram was born [event time] in June [cosmic time]'.

Trouble (Vikram's illness, the gang-rape) is the raw material from which plot is woven. Until there is a breach in the humdrum of everyday life, from what we expected to happen (and from what does happen, day in, day out), there is no story (Bruner, 1986). In the illness narrative, the focus of trouble is death, disability, disfigurement, distress, intractable pain, loss of freedom, or social stigma. The essence of the illness narrative is how well or how badly health professionals, caregivers and patients evade or face up to these adversities – and this, of course, depends on their character. Heroes are made when individuals tackle their own illness-related troubles or step in (courageously, determinedly, selflessly) to help others out of theirs. The villain is he who maliciously exacerbates trouble, or she whose slothful inaction delays restitution. As Aristotle perceptively pointed out, most people are neither exceptionally virtuous nor wholly

---

[1] In this book, I use the terms 'story' and 'narrative' interchangeably. I acknowledge that scholars have filled volumes with philosophical small print on the subtle differences between them.

wicked. Rather, 'trouble' will bring out the best – or the worst – in an otherwise unremarkable individual.

Emplotment is the use of literary devices to align events and link them through the purposeful actions of characters, thereby getting our heroes and villains in and out of trouble, and to show (at least implicitly) whose fault it all was. Trouble, and the response to it, is conveyed through literary tropes such as repetition, metaphor, irony, surprise, and so on.[2] There may be a period of suspense in which we, the audience, do not know how bad the impact of the trouble will be (the 'cliffhanger' – what one writer (Mattingly, 1998) has described as 'the emotionally charged moment of not-knowing'). But as Aristotle himself made clear, dramatic suspense is often a blunt instrument in the literary world, and a good plot is usually achieved through subtler tropes (Aristotle, 1996b).

In the excerpt at the beginning of this chapter, for example, Vikram's father uses the word 'normal' six times – to refer variously to his son's birth, his first few minutes of life, the milk he was fed, and the nature and frequency of his early cough. As the story unfolds, expressions depicting Vikram as not-ill ('normal', 'common', 'okay', comparable to his not-ill brother) gradually give way to those depicting Vikram as ill ('not normal', 'really bad', 'his problem'), until it becomes clear that a family catastrophe (the diagnosis of Vikram's major heart defect) is unavoidable – a state of affairs that Aristotle called recognition (*anagnorisis* – the change from ignorance to knowledge; the 'aha' moment in the story). But even at the outset, there is a hint of concern – the seeds of trouble. As we read the story fragment, we are repeatedly and rhetorically pulled between 'Vikram as not-ill' and 'Vikram as ill', and in this way the narrator conveys something of the anxiety and confusion that he and his wife felt before the definitive diagnosis was made.

Aristotle described a number of genres for plots in ancient Greece – chiefly tragedy, comedy and epic. Most Hollywood plots can be classified as adventure (the good guy overcomes trouble to win a reward), romance (the good guy gets the girl), irony (the self-styled hero is exposed as a fool)

---

[2] Aristotle described three 'master tropes' – metaphor (depicting the unfamiliar by reference to the familiar, as in 'surfing the Internet'), metonym (implicating one feature with another feature that is contiguous in time or space, as in 'the Crown' to indicate the monarch who wears it) and synecdoche (depicting the whole by reference to a part, as in 'Give us this day our daily bread', where 'bread' represents food in general). A fourth trope, irony (the use of words to express something different from, and often opposite to, their literal meaning, as in the wonderful nickname 'Totty' – a slang term for cheap and sexy – given by a group of schoolboys to a particularly stern and charmless female teacher in Alan Bennett's *The History Boys*), was added by medieval scholars (Burke, 1945).

or melodrama (a charged battle between good and evil, usually with a climactic battle towards the end). Arthur Frank, a professor of sociology who has written movingly about his own serious illnesses (Frank, 1991, 1995), divides illness narratives into four broad genres:

- restitution (the doctor-hero accurately diagnoses and treats the illness and/or the patient-hero successfully navigates a complex system of care to achieve the desired cure)
- tragedy (the doctor-hero does his or her best but the patient nevertheless succumbs – or, perhaps, the patient-hero struggles unsuccessfully to survive and be heard in the face of medical incompetence or insensitivity)
- quest (the patient-hero embarks on a journey to find meaning and purpose in his or her incurable illness)
- chaos (the story is incoherent, unsatisfying, and does not make sense) (Frank, 1995).

Vikram's father's narrative, which has begun as tragedy, could yet develop into either restitution (if his son's heart condition is successfully treated) or a more profound tragedy (if it isn't). The use of comedy in illness narratives is surprisingly common, especially when people are describing a brush with an inefficient healthcare system ('they said "We're wheeling you down for your operation, Mr Brown, as we've finally found your notes", and I said, "My name's Smith actually; Brown died in the night"'). The use of humorous tropes sublimates the anxiety about a 'near-miss' medical mishap, and also effectively highlights the absurdity of disorganisation and staff indifference when human life hangs in the balance.

Context is the concrete here-and-now of the story being told. A parent's narrative about his infant with ventricular septal defect isn't about congenital heart disease in general, but about *this* family living in this house, at this time, and coping – or failing to cope – with this child, cared for by this medical system. Illness is the trouble that throws a spanner in the works – but in order to understand the illness, we need also to understand the 'works' into which the spanner is thrown.

'A central difficulty with clinical renderings of patient sufferings is that in their abstractness, the world of the patient is left out. This world is above all a practical and moral one in which patients have life projects and everyday concerns, things 'at stake'. What comes to be 'at stake' for any individual

> depends, in part, on the local moral world the patient inhabits. Illness . . .
> creates a 'resistance' which hinders or prevents the sufferer from carrying out
> plans and projects.'
>
> (Mattingly, 1998)

There is another important dimension to context. All narratives, although on one level personal and specific, are on another level a reflection of a particular society with a particular set of norms and values. For example, Vikram's father's story about his son's delayed diagnosis is also a story about the responsibility of the GP as gatekeeper to specialist care. In a different healthcare system in a different country, Vikram would have been taken directly to a paediatrician. In yet another country, his first encounter might have been with a witch doctor. Those of us who work as GPs in the UK face a huge challenge – to detect early signs of serious illness when it presents non-specifically (that is, with symptoms that also occur very commonly in not-ill patients).[3]

Illness narratives convey important cultural messages about appropriate social roles (how should a good doctor, a good family member or a good citizen behave towards a person with this sort of illness?) and about what to do in particular circumstances (for example, after childbirth, or when newly diagnosed with epilepsy). Katherine Montgomery Hunter, a professor of literature who spent many years doing fieldwork in a hospital, has demonstrated that the ritualistic exchange of stories by doctors in the 'grand round' is a critical way of passing on both scientific knowledge and

---

[3] Although some missed diagnoses can be attributable to genuine clinical failure (doctors, after all, are human), there is an interesting literature from Bayesian statistics on the predictive value of different clinical signs when working in a population of not-very-sick individuals. Back in 1991, Morley and colleagues studied over a thousand sick and not-so-sick babies in hospital and primary care. They checked various symptoms and signs and correlated these with four grades of illness severity. Most symptoms (slow feeding, sweating, crying, cough, rash, and so on) were associated to some extent or other with all grades of illness. Only four symptoms were never reported in infants who turned out not to be sick: a fluid intake less than a third of normal, convulsions, frank blood in the stools, and bile-stained vomiting (Morley *et al.*, 1991). From a Bayesian perspective, it is astonishing how much serious illness *is* detected promptly by GPs and how many not-ill infants are spared the traumas of hospital referral. Overall, generalist care is both more effective and more cost-effective than providing specialist investigations and treatment to the not-ill, not-yet-ill, or not-very-ill (Baicker and Chandra, 2004). The nature of the judgements that allow GPs, most of the time, successfully to extract the 'seriously ill' needles from the haystacks of non-specific presentations is a topic that I have addressed elsewhere in a paper on intuition in general practice (Greenhalgh, 2002).

professional norms and values (Hunter, 1991), a theme to which I shall return in Chapter Six (Stories and ethics).

The academic literature on narrative contains a number of different viewpoints on what narrative *is*. Consider, for example, three contrasting views:

1 *The referential (mimetic) perspective.* Narrative (storytelling) is a person's report on what happened. In the words of sociolinguist William Labov, whose narrative-based research from the 1950s is still widely cited, narrative is 'the recapitulation of past experience' by means of an account consisting of 'at least two past tense event clauses where the order of the clauses represents the order of events' (Labov, 1982). The referential perspective is considered by many academics to be somewhat outdated, but it is still very much part of the medical tradition – the doctor or nurse 'takes a history' (i.e. asks questions of the patient and then writes down the 'facts'). Anthropologists have demonstrated that medical students get progressively less adept at capturing the key elements of a person's illness narrative as they progress from Year 1 to Year 3 of their clinical medical training (Good, 1994). This is not to say that they get worse at recording the 'facts', but (perhaps) that their pursuit of a faithful representation of events suppresses key literary elements (such as a patient's choice of metaphor) that could inform a diagnosis or therapeutic choice, and it also makes them less able to contribute to a transformative telling (see below).

2 *The transformative (anti-mimetic) perspective.* Narrative does not merely report what happened, but in some way it also changes it. Most importantly, an autobiographical narrative does not merely describe the self – it *creates* that self. In Vikram's father's narrative of the trips to and from the primary healthcare team, Vikram is presented as a victim (vulnerable and helpless as he is in the face of medical reassurances that will be revisited in retrospect), and he himself is presented as a devoted father who becomes a hero through his dogged insistence that his child must be re-examined.

   Many writers have emphasised the critical importance of storytelling in the creation of identity – we tell stories about ourselves (and others like us) in order to affirm, and sometimes to change, *who* we are (Bruner, 1990; Riessman, 1990; Mishler, 1999; Holstein & Gubrium, 2000). The illness narrative not only describes the experience of suffering and depicts efforts to overcome or make sense of it – it also reframes or reaffirms the narrator's identity (Kleinmann, 1988; Riessman, 1990; Mattingly & Garro, 2000). I shall discuss this theme in more detail in Chapter Two (Stories and healing).

3 *The performative perspective.* Narrative is not merely a looking back at action, but *is itself an action.* For example, the illness narrative might be viewed as a play enacted on the 'stage' of the consulting room (a performative narrative) – a theme explored particularly in the fieldwork and theoretical approach of US anthropologist Cheryl Mattingly (Mattingly, 1998). The notion of performative narrative was also used by Erving Goffman in his seminal work on the construction of the self. Social actors, he claimed, stage performances of desirable selves to preserve face in situations of difficulty, such as chronic illness. Talk is not primarily about giving information to a recipient, but about the staging of dramas to an audience (Goffman, 1981). Those interested in the performative framing of narrative should also see Victor Turner's work on social performance (Turner, 1986) and Clifford Geertz's discussion of action as text (Geertz, 1988). In Chapter Four (Stories and organisations) I apply the concept of performative narrative to the challenge of organisational change, rejecting mechanical plan–do–study–act cycles in favour of the more enticing metaphor of social drama.

Clinicians who first learned to evaluate medical texts according to the rules of evidence-based practice (in which all written sources are classified according to a strict quality hierarchy) often hold the view that nothing ranks below story – especially the raw, unverified narrative of the patient's own words – in the hierarchy of evidence. Such individuals, even those who resist this hierarchy, often seek a comparable set of criteria to check the 'worth' of an illness narrative. I have already argued that narrative truth is fundamentally different from scientific truth, but where does this leave us in practice? A number of authors have attempted to address the quality of the illness narrative from a theoretical standpoint, and several potential criteria (listed below) are worth considering further. The story told by Vikram's father on page 3 was first collected as part of a research project (see www.dipex.org.uk), and was certainly never intended to be evaluated as a piece of literature. Nevertheless, it meets a number of criteria of a 'good story', which are listed below.

Aesthetic appeal – i.e. the story is pleasing to hear and recount, and demonstrates a kind of internal harmony. Aristotle in ancient times and philosopher Kenneth Burke in the twentieth century (among many others) emphasised the importance of achieving a balance between the different elements in the story (characters, plot, context, actions, trouble, and so on) (Burke, 1945; Aristotle, 1996b). The artistic merit of a story is a central preoccupation of literary criticism and mostly beyond the scope of this book, but as Launer suggests, we can all spot a good story in clinical practice, just as we can in the arts (Launer, 2002). The patient who makes a minor illness into a melodrama induces less sympathy than they might otherwise have gained. One who inserts too much detail will be viewed as a 'poor historian' (and in medicine's rather shameful past, might have been formally labelled as such on the front of their medical record). But – and perhaps I should present this statement as a research hypothesis, since I have no proof that it is the case – the patient whose story is seen as genuinely touching, humorous, ironic or otherwise appealing can anticipate a corresponding increase in the doctor or nurse's engagement and motivation to help. We feel the more for Vikram's father because of the unassuming and appealing way in which he presents his unfolding family tragedy.

Coherence – i.e. the story is clear and the succession of events and actions makes a logical whole; it does not contain inherent muddles or puzzles. One aspect of coherence is *moral order*, namely that there is a point to the story that makes moral sense, even if the characters lack virtue and the ending is tragic (Ricoeur, 1984). All too commonly the illness story as heard by doctors and therapists is the 'chaos' or 'heartsink' narrative that is incoherent and deeply unsatisfying all round – not only is there no discernible plot, but no one is sure which character is doing what, or with what motive (Frank, 1995; Bligh, 1999; Launer, 2002). But the chaos narrative, by its very discordance, tells us something important – about which more in Chapter Two (Stories and healing). Vikram's father's story, of which only the first instalment is reproduced here, achieves a satisfying (though tragic) coherence in the last line when we are told the definitive diagnosis. Having seen the main character swing uneasily between 'ill' and 'not-ill', we (the readers of and listeners to the story) are relieved of our uncertainty by this final sentence, and can now move on to the second phase of the action in which, hopefully, Vikram starts to get better.

Authenticity – i.e. the credibility of the story. This is comparable to, but not the same as, scientific validity. We do not condemn a fairy story for being fanciful, but we would object if it didn't behave as a fairy story should. Those of us who are parents find Vikram's father's story credible because we can identify with the repeated trips made to the GP with a sick child, and the power-charged negotiations about how ill he is or isn't. Those of us who are health professionals find it credible because this story rings true for us in our clinical role, resonating subconsciously with a dose of misplaced reassurance that we ourselves have dished out in the past. Even if we have never been in a directly comparable situation ourselves, the story is still authentic as something that *could* happen to someone like us, in a situation like ours. As Aristotle put it, *'it is not the function of the poet to relate what has happened, but what may happen – what is possible according to the law of probability or necessity'* (Aristotle, 1996b).

> *'A good story and a well-formed argument are different natural kinds. Both can be used as a means for convincing another. Yet what they convince of is fundamentally different: arguments convince of their truth, stories of their lifelikeness. The one verifies by eventual appeal to procedures for establishing formal and empirical truth. The other establishes its truth by verisimilitude.'*
>
> (Bruner, 1986)

Reportability – i.e. the 'so what' value. If in a crowded room we overhear a story about a death, or a near-miss death, we stop and listen. Death is the ultimate reportable event – the opposite to something that doesn't matter (and about which, therefore, there is no story). Dramatic tension in books and films is very often about a death that might be avoided (e.g. if Superman can get there soon enough). Labov has suggested that the failed narrative is the one that leaves the listener wondering why the story was told at all (Labov, 1982). Vikram's story is highly reportable because it is the ultimate life-in-the-balance narrative. Vikram is about as young, innocent and full of hope as a human character could be. His illness – what my mother would have called a 'hole in the heart' – is potentially catastrophic (and also symbolically so, the heart being the fount of Vikram's life-blood metaphorically as well as physiologically).

In a medical encounter, serious illness is indisputably reportable, but trivial symptoms are traditionally considered less so ('a waste of the doctor's time'). As medical science increasingly seeks to detect potentially serious diseases at an early (treatable) stage, there have been some interesting campaigns to increase public and professional perceptions about the reportability of seemingly inconsequential symptoms, such as twinges of chest pain, coughs that don't settle, and rashes that fail to blanche on pressure. To cite a concrete example, a heart attack patient arriving at hospital between 4 and 12 hours after the onset of chest pain is three times as likely to die as one arriving within an hour of that onset, yet the average time patients take to call for help is around 4 hours. Delay in seeking help is much more likely if the symptoms are vague and undramatic, and mass media campaigns have had minimal short-term and no long-term impact on delay (Penny, 2001). The lack of success of such campaigns is perhaps attributable to something hard-wired in us as storytellers and story-listeners – if there is no obvious danger, we simply don't bother to report to the doctor.

Persuasiveness. Related to reportability is the notion that narrative is rhetorical – that is, that a key purpose of narrative is not merely to entertain the listener or convey information, but to persuade them of one's own perspective on something. The patient who brings a story of pain seeks not merely to receive physical treatment, but also to formalise and legitimise their suffering through the doctor's (or nurse's) bearing witness to the story (Good *et al.*, 1994). Vikram's father's negotiations with the GP about the significance (and thus the reportability) of his child's cough constitutes an interesting story-within-a-story. Would the parent-hero succeed in his attempt to persuade the powerful, knowledge-rich GP to accept his version of reality (that Vikram was ill) over the previously given professional assertion that Vikram was *not* ill?

'People do not tell their stories in a vacuum. They must fight (be good rhetoricians or debaters) to tell their story and to have it more or less accepted, authorized, or taken up by others. They try to control the circumstances of its hearing and, to some degree, of its interpretation. But the telling is an interaction in which the audience (or interlocutor) actively shapes the telling and the teller – indeed, in which more than one (story)teller is active at once, and each shapes the other in an ongoing contest.'

(Kirmayer, 2000)

Whilst it can be a useful exercise to draw on literary theory when considering whether a particular illness narrative is a 'good' one, other writers have suggested a much more pragmatic definition in terms of how *useful* the story is in achieving particular ends for the sick person (such as reaching a diagnosis or achieving a return to work) (Launer, 2002). A story might be useful for the patient but less useful for the practitioner or third parties (the obvious example being the 50-minute unburdening narrative on a Monday morning that makes the patient feel better but leaves the doctor exhausted and running late[4]). In contrast, a useful story for the doctor might be one that leads to prompt diagnosis or an evidence-based treatment protocol!

The usefulness (or fitness for purpose) of an illness narrative has a number of dimensions.

1 *Explanatory value* – i.e. it helps the patient to explain, articulate and understand what is happening to them (Greenhalgh & Hurwitz, 1999), a process I shall expand upon in Chapter Two (Stories and healing).
2 *Diagnostic and therapeutic value* – i.e. it helps the clinician to match what is happening to this patient against 'narrative scripts' of diseases and treatment protocols (Kleinmann, 1988; Cox, 2001). Indeed, an extreme view might be that the 'good illness narrative' can be mapped to a formal disease taxonomy and coded accordingly on the computer. However, as I discuss in Chapter Two (see in particular the discussion about Bakhtin on page 21), the instrumental use of the illness narrative by doctors in traditional diagnostic roles raises interesting philosophical questions.
3 *Illuminative value* – i.e. even when it fails to point clearly to a preferred course of action, the illness narrative can highlight the unknowns, the practical tensions and the moral ambiguities that the patient is faced with (and which the clinician is being asked to share) (Rubin, 2002). Chapter Six (Stories and ethics) explores this theme in more detail.
4 *Transformative value* – i.e. it generates new meaning and may, for example, allow a sad, tired, hopeless or uncaring story to become a story that is more vigorous, hopeful or caring. An individual's illness

[4] In these days of the 'narrative turn' in medicine, and notwithstanding the theoretical points I make in Chapter Two, it is worth reflecting on the lengthy, repetitive and compulsively told illness narrative, into which the doctor is reluctantly drawn, and which seems to do neither party much good. Psychoanalysts would have a different interpretation, but my clinical experience suggests that good medicine does not equate to uncritical and timeless 'listenership'. There is a literary parallel here, illustrated by Adam Zachary Newton's commentary on Coleridge's *Rime of the Ancient Mariner*, in which the Wedding Guest, Hermit and various interlocutors are drawn into the grip of the Mariner's obsessive story ('He cannot choose but hear'). The Mariner, tellingly, is aware that he is condemned continually to repeat his own story ('Since then, at an uncertain hour/ The agony returns/ Until my ghastly tale is told / The heart within me burns') – yet recounting it to successive captive audiences brings no long-term catharsis (Newton, 1995).

narrative is not merely a story about the self and the illness – it is a dynamic and discursive *shaping* of that self in the face of illness (Riessman, 1990; Mishler, 1999). If (and to the extent that) the transformative narrative is about a changed and better self, the story both describes and creates appropriate virtues such as strength, courage, coping or acquiescence (about which more in Chapter Six). This, of course, is the foundation on which 'talking therapies' of their various kinds (*see* Chapter Two) are built.

To summarise the main points of this chapter, a narrative is a chronological account of purposeful action by people in the face of (or with a view to causing) trouble, set in a particular real or imaginary context. It is inherently non-linear in that key structuring devices are surprise, suspense and 'twists in the plot', achieved through literary tropes such as repetition, imagery and metaphor. 'Narrative truth' is not about scientific accuracy but about conveying something of the human condition through an appeal to emotions. A good illness narrative has literary features: it is artistically appealing, coherent, authentic, reportable and persuasive. But such a narrative may also have practical qualities: it effectively conveys and explains the subjective experience of illness; it aids diagnosis; it suggests therapeutic choices; it illuminates practical and moral ambiguities; and finally, through its construction, it transforms both the sufferer and the experience of suffering.

Although there is no doubt that medicine has taken a 'narrative turn', remarkably few illness narratives (even those that hit the bestseller list) have exceptional literary qualities. In reality, many illness narratives remain unheard, and many more fail to illuminate, inform, heal or transform the experience that they describe. Therein lies the challenge for clinicians – and I guess that is why I wrote this book. In the next chapter (Stories and healing), I consider the potential for narrative to contribute to the healing process, and the role of the health professional as listener. In Chapter Three (Stories and learning), I describe a research project of my own in which my team applied the narrative principles to the education of health advocates and patients. In Chapter Four (Stories and organisations), I consider organisational narratives as a window to more general insights about how healthcare organisations work and how we might try to change them. In Chapter Five (Stories and research), I describe how narrative techniques can be used when researching the illness experience and the organisation and delivery of healthcare, and I suggest some provisional ways of defining and judging quality in such research. In Chapter Six (Stories and ethics), I return to the question of how the story form helps us to address moral questions of 'what to do' and 'who to be'. This final chapter also explores how literature can illuminate ethical issues that are inaccessible by other means, and considers the ethical challenges of collecting and using stories in research, teaching and quality improvement.

Chapter Two

Stories and healing

Dr Patel:	Hello Mrs Dunn, what can I do for you?
Mrs Dunn:	[pause] To be honest I'm not sure. Tired all the time, this and that.
Dr Patel:	Mmm?
Mrs Dunn:	[silent]
Dr Patel:	How's the family?
Mrs Dunn:	Oh, so-so. [another pause]
Dr Patel:	Is this a routine asthma check?
Mrs Dunn:	[shakes head] I know I'm due for that but . . .
Dr Patel:	. . . Yes, you are. We changed your inhalers last time, didn't we? And I asked you to see the nurse.
Mrs Dunn:	[looking down] I didn't keep that appointment. I wasn't feeling well. . . .
Dr Patel:	Uh-huh?
Mrs Dunn:	. . . No. I'd hurt my eye.
Dr Patel:	Oh yes?
Mrs Dunn:	Just a bit of bruising, nothing too serious. It's better now.
Dr Patel:	[putting his pen down and looking at her] Tell me more.
Mrs Dunn:	[cries]
Dr Patel:	Did anyone hit you?
Mrs Dunn:	[pause] Only the once . . .

A typical personal narrative set out in print (as in an autobiography, or the transcript of Vikram's father's story on page 3) reads as a monologue – a stream of text initiated and sustained by the narrator, created by him or her alone, and reproduced verbatim by the person reading it out. But real (oral) narrative is rarely like that. 'Once upon a time there was a king . . .' you might begin, and you can soon anticipate an interruption by your listener: 'Was he a good king? Did he have a queen?'. In reality, your story will not be a faithful reproduction of the text in the story book, but an *interactional narrative* between you and your listener. This is the stuff of clinical consultations, with the various interjections such as 'uh-huh', 'mmm', 'tell me more about that' and even 'look here, we've only got seven minutes' helping to shape the patient's story. Whilst most narrative theorists agree that teller–listener interaction influences an unfolding story (Labov, for example, emphasised the importance of the listener's response in designating the reportability of the narrative) (Labov, 1982), simply acknowledging this influence is very different from suggesting that interaction is the fundamental essence of narrative.

Interactional narrative – narrative as co-constructed by the narrator and the listener – is an example of the transformative perspective (*see* page 13). Whereas Labov's structural approach to narrative separates the reporting of events from their evaluation (as in 'he stole my bag; it was a dreadful thing to do'), most contemporary narrative theorists argue that there is no reporting of trouble without its interpretation, and that reporting is a creative act (Gwyn, 2002). Furthermore, reporting and interpretation constitute a *dialogue*, not a monologue.

This principle is illustrated in the fragment from a consultation between a patient (Mrs Dunn) and her GP (Dr Patel) on the previous page, which is fictitious but based on a real encounter. At the beginning of the consultation, Mrs Dunn appears lost for words. Dr Patel invites her to tell her story but she has, it seems, no clear story to recount. Her non-specific symptom (tiredness) is linked with a general sense of confusion about associated events ('this and that'). The GP offers a nudge ('Mmm?') and then a prompt ('How's the family?'), to which she responds in a poignantly non-committal way. The GP then attempts to lead the narrative along the lines of a routine biomedical check-up (in this case, for asthma), but Mrs Dunn inserts a cue ('I didn't keep that appointment [because] I wasn't feeling well'), which indicates that she does not intend this to be a straightforward 'check-up' narrative. Indeed, Mrs Dunn's implication that not feeling well required her to miss the asthma check-up suggests quite explicitly that the illness to be attended to was not asthma. The doctor picks up on the cue ('Uh-huh?') and, using various follow-up prompts ('Oh yes?' and 'Tell me more'), supports the patient in constructing the beginnings of a very different narrative – that of domestic violence.

In this example, Dr Patel is neither conventionally 'directive' (asking a series of questions which the patient is expected to answer) nor con-ventionally 'non-directive' (allowing the patient to make every move in the conversation). Towards the end of the excerpt, for example, he asks very directly, 'Did anyone hit you?', a question which Mrs Dunn appears not to resent (indeed, according to qualitative research studies on the topic, she probably welcomes being asked) (Jewkes, 2002). Until we reach what Labov (1982) would call the maximally reportable event – that Mrs Dunn has been hit – the doctor has contributed little to the conversation except 'Uh-huh?'! Yet his role has been far from passive. This is not non-directive consulting but interactional narrative, a crucial feature of which is perhaps simple curiosity – wanting to know (and caring about) the next part of the story (Launer, 2002).

The Russian philosopher and linguist Mikhail Bakhtin, who began writing at around the time of the Russian revolution, made a key contribution to narrative theory with his claim that all text is dialogical. What he meant by this was that every utterance – even 'uh-huh' – is made in response to (or anticipation of) some other utterance. The audience, claimed Bakhtin, is centrally involved in creating the meaning of the texts they read or hear. Without an audience, the text has no meaning.

> *'Human thought becomes genuine thought, that is, an idea, only under conditions of living contact with another and alien thought, a thought embodied in someone else's voice.'*
>
> (Bakhtin, 1984)

In Bakhtin's view, the role of the listener is not merely to absorb a story passively, but to provide a separate perspective – something which soci-ologist Arthur Frank describes as *critical distance* (Frank, 1998). Drawing on Bakhtin, Frank takes issue with conventional biomedical perspectives on patients' stories (see, for example, *The Illness Narratives*) (Kleinmann, 1988), in which doctors are encouraged to use listening as a diagnostic tool for extracting information that can contribute to a problem-solving sequence. In such an approach, he claims, *'the [patient] remains the object of the professional's privileged subjectivity: there is no relationship in the sense of reciprocated feeling for one another'* (Frank, 1998). But in a Bakhtinian framing of clinical interaction, the role of the clinician is to provide the subjective 'otherness' for an interactional narrative in which the patient will construct, and make sense of, his or her illness narrative.

In the exchange on page 19, Dr Patel did not 'take a history' of domestic violence using conventional diagnostic questions. Indeed, in the remainder of this consultation (not shown) he was careful not to ask any more direct questions about the domestic incident. The doctor's input was both less and more than that of a conventional diagnostician – he provided the curiosity and critical distance that allowed the patient to construct the first fragment of her painful and shocking story. Over the next few months, and within the protected confines of the consulting room, Mrs Dunn's domestic violence story unfolded gradually, alongside her asthma narrative and her wife-and-mother narrative. All three were subtly woven into a wider tapestry of seemingly inconsequential story fragments – her young daughter's hay fever, her son's eczema – that make up the bread and butter of general practice consultations (and which, as Michael Balint's meticulous research on the nature of general practice demonstrated, are often the presenting complaint that gets the patient through the door with his or her 'hidden agenda') (Balint, 1959).

On page 11 I introduced Jerome Bruner's notion of the narrative truth derived from a good story as distinct from the logico-deductive truth derived from scientific method. As I shall argue later in this chapter, the rigorous and conscientious application of logico-deductive truths (as in evidence-based medicine) is undeniably a critical dimension of good clinical care. Equally critical, however, is the recognition of narrative truth – the empathetic bearing of witness to the patient's story, and especially to his or her account of personal trouble and heroic efforts to face and resolve it. This witness-bearing is a complex exercise in inter-subjectivity which Frank (with deliberate irony) has called 'just listening' (Frank, 1998).

'Just listening' encompasses not only the various forms of talking therapy offered to those with distress or mental illness, but also the intermittent dialogue of long-term continuing care for patients with chronic illness, and the especially intimate story shared with a patient who is, or might soon be, dying. The accumulation of (often brief and disjointed) clinician–patient encounters over time constitutes above all else 'just listening' to an unfolding restitution, tragedy or quest narrative (*see* page 6). If the chronic illness story unfolds in what Frank would call a chaos narrative, 'just listening' provides the opportunity for both parties to co-construct a new narrative that holds some meaning for the patient and can begin to unfold for better or worse, but as a story should. The GP who invites the patient to 'come and see me again in a couple of weeks to tell me how you're getting on', and the cancer nurse who offers to 'pop in when I'm next passing', have recognised that the central purpose of the encounter is not for a diagnosis, a procedure or a prescription – but simply, and crucially, for another instalment in the story.

As I implied in my footnote on page 13, and as illustrated by Dr Patel's interjections in the example on page 19, 'just listening' to a chaos narrative is a complex skill that is not merely being present at the pouring out of trouble. The American physician and narratologist Rita Charon has developed both a theory and a practical training for 'just listening'. In her words, *'The effective practice of medicine requires narrative competence, that is the ability to acknowledge, absorb, interpret and act on the stories and plights of others'* (Charon, 2001).

Charon's notion of narrative competence goes beyond the skills required in conventional models of medical consulting such as 'concord-ance' (Royal Pharmaceutical Society of Great Britain, 1997) or 'shared decision making' (Towle & Godolphin, 1999). She argues at a higher level of abstraction – that the practice of medicine is comparable to reading (that is, immersion in and interpretation of) a text. The link is not merely logical (sickness calls forth stories, so the doctor must be able to hear and understand them), but also allegorical (sickness *is* a text that must be read). As I shall argue in more detail in Chapter Six, both literature and medicine are fundamentally about ethical choices – that is, about *what best to do* in the face of trouble.

'Literature's narrative ethics examines the reciprocal responsibilities incurred by the writer who encodes thoughts and feelings into language and by the reader who rescues from words their secrets. Writer and reader (or teller and listener) develop deep powers and daring intimacies as they meet in text, for the writer, however cannily or uncannily, reveals aspects of the self while the reader, with whatever skill is available, penetrates the text toward that which put it in motion.'

(Charon, 2001)

Similarly, the 'just listening' of the healing relationship requires the development of a shared ethical perspective, based on a common – although, crucially, not identical – reading of the situation and context.

> '*The conversation one has with another – the patient, the family, the nurse, the intern – rests on the intersubjective pact, that is, the agreement that one is not completely alone in interpreting this construction of reality. One stands oneself as a sign for the other, making room in the reasoning, with risk and utter trust, for the interpretation offered by another. In the clinical world, of course, such pacts are complicated by and implicated in the vulnerability of illness, the power asymmetries in hospitals, and the little time there usually is in which to act.*'
>
> (Charon, 2001)

Like most physicians, Professor Charon spends much of her time caring for patients with heart failure, diabetes and other medical conditions that have strict diagnostic criteria and for which there are evidence-based management guidelines. How does her PhD in English literature enable her to improve clinical outcomes in these patients above and beyond what any 'evidence-based' clinician might achieve? My own answer is that the science of evidence-based medicine (EBM), fine and rigorous though it is, was built on a myth – that the judgements required in clinical practice are fundamentally technical ones, achieved purely through the skilled application of evidence-based medicine's tools of the trade (procedures, investigations and therapeutic protocols). According to this view of reality, quality in clinical medicine can be assured by the scientific robustness of the recommendations and protocols, and the technical precision with which they are applied to each case.

In some clinical situations, this myth approximates so closely to reality that it is entirely appropriate to work on the assumption that patients get ill, consult their physicians, take their medicine, have operations, receive nursing care and physiotherapy, get better or worse, and at some stage die in an entirely clockwork universe whose behaviour is fathomable and predictable so long as the right tests are ordered and the right treatment algorithm is applied. But where do Mrs Dunn and her doctor (*see* page 19) fit into such a universe? In a different version of this consultation – one that was not merely evidence-based but naively evidence-driven – Dr Patel would have followed the pop-up prompt on his computer screen that told him Mrs Dunn's blood pressure was overdue for checking. In doing so, he would have obtained a clinically important item of data at the expense of the trust we see being built through the subtle exchange of 'uh-huhs' and 'this and thats' in the consultation fragment on page 19.

He would also have failed to incur the ethical obligation that we see emerging when, at the end of this stop-start exchange, Mrs Dunn's shameful secret is disclosed. Such trade-offs will never be quantifiable, but Scandinavian GP Karl-Edward Rudebeck (cited in Iona Heath's excellent monograph *The Mystery of General Practice*, a previous publication in the John Fry monograph series) (Heath, 1997) has argued passionately that general practice must not be pushed into *'defining itself at its own margins, leaving its very centre, its specific priorities, unfathomed by both critics and spokesmen.'*

Back in the 1970s, one of England's first professors of general practice, Marshall Marinker, penned a satirical critique of specialist medicine in the *Journal of the Royal College of General Practitioners*. In it he argued somewhat cynically that the key task of specialists is to *'distinguish the clear message of the disease from the interfering noise of the patient as a person'* (Marinker, 1978), and that they achieve this by deliberately excluding (indeed, by working within a professional jargon that is designed to exclude) aspects of the patient's illness experience that do not fit textbook models of diseases.[5] More recently, the New Zealand professor of family medicine, J Campbell Murdoch, has argued that whereas textbook perspectives on general practice are generally built around various medical and quasi-medical categories (diseases, diagnoses, families, communities, and so on), such a taxonomy is hard to spot in the real-life experience of primary healthcare, where categories of 'not sick', 'not yet sick' and 'inexplicably sick' are needed at least as much as 'definitely sick'. In such a universe, the dominant frames are poverty, exclusion, addiction, loneliness, rejection, failure and, above all, uncertainty (Murdoch, 1997). In this latter world, the patient's story – fragmented, incomplete and inconsistent as it is – is often a more helpful unit of analysis than the textbook diagnostic category or evidence-based management protocol (Launer, 2002).

As medicine shifts its core business from the treatment of acute illnesses to the long-term management of chronic ones, as more and more evidence accumulates of the contribution of inequalities (of income, information, language, social capital, access to services, and so on) to adverse health outcomes (Marmot, 2003), and as clinical judgement is increasingly shown to be a fundamentally interpretive rather than logico-deductive

---

[5] Elliot Mishler, drawing on the work of critical theorist Jurgen Habermas, has developed a more sophisticated theoretical model of 'distinguishing the clear message of the disease' from the 'interfering noise of the patient as a person'. His distinction is between the 'Voice of Medicine' and the 'Voice of the Lifeworld', and is discussed further in Chapter Five (page 75) when I consider narrative approaches to research.

process (Hamm, 2003), the fracture points of evidence-based medicine's clockwork universe become more clearly exposed. Notwithstanding the value of the randomised controlled trial, the multiple regression analysis and the quality-adjusted life-year (all of which I am completely signed up to, in their place), the assiduous pursuit of the 'clear message of the disease' and the attempt to treat that disease in an entirely standardised and algorithm-driven way is becoming an increasingly inappropriate goal in both primary and secondary healthcare.

I would be entirely happy, however, if Dr Patel chose to draw upon evidence-based medicine in his efforts to help Mrs Dunn to deal as best she can with the traumas in her life. Indeed, I would venture to suggest that, having heard enough of Mrs Dunn's story to fit it with the 'illness script' of domestic violence (Cox, 2001), I would be disappointed if Dr Patel failed to incorporate the important findings from research studies that are summarised in the leading British EBM textbook *Clinical Evidence* in a section (sandwiched between 'Diarrhoea' and 'Dysmenorrhoea') entitled 'Domestic violence towards women' (Klevens & Sadowski, 2005). Difficult though randomised controlled trials must be in this field of enquiry, several have been done. Talking therapies alone seem to have little impact on re-abuse, but advocacy (defined in this context as *'providing information to a client on her legal, medical, and financial options; facilitating her access to and use of community resources such as shelters, counselling, and protection orders; accessing and mobilising her natural support networks; assisting in goal setting and making choices; validating her feelings of being victimised; and providing emotional support'*) and safety planning (*'helping participants to identify behaviours that might signal increased danger and prepare, ahead of time, codes of communication with family or friends, as well as needed documents, keys, and clothing should a quick exit become necessary'*) both significantly reduce the incidence of re-abuse.

I have quoted extensively from *Clinical Evidence* in this example to illustrate that, in my view, 'just listening' (the provision of a Bakhtinian 'otherness') is not an excuse to throw the baby out with the bathwater. Faced with a patient with acute chest pain, few clinicians would 'just listen'. We can do better than 'just listen' to the victims of domestic violence, too. But as the exchange between Mrs Dunn and her doctor on page 19 shows, 'just listening' was what set the stage for the all-important disclosure. In another of his timeless treatises, *Rhetoric*, Aristotle wrote that one of the key skills of argumentation (which he, like many ancient Greeks, viewed as a highly scholarly activity) is the imaginative and intuitive decision about *where to begin* (Aristotle, 2005). Philosopher

Alasdair MacIntyre makes a similar point in his book *After Virtue* in relation to ethical judgements. The story (for our purposes, the patient's rather than the doctor's version of the illness narrative) allows the ethicist to identify that most fundamental precursor of the ethical decision – the nature of the problem and where to begin. I shall discuss MacIntyre's work further in Chapter Six, but let us now return to Mrs Dunn. Had Dr Patel begun his evidence-based decision making at the obvious place (with asthma or hypertension), he would have short-changed his patient. Because he placed high priority on the quality of the interactional narrative, and was sensitive to the new story that was tentatively emerging, he discovered the starting point at which his patient – probably unconsciously – sought to begin their dialogue.

To return to my question about how a scholarly understanding of literature helps Rita Charon in her work as a doctor, let me quote from a chapter she wrote recently for a book I co-edited. She described a patient with complex needs – poor, depressed, living alone, with multiple medical problems including intractable back pain and atrial fibrillation on anti-coagulants, and communicating through an interpreter.

'The woman's dense depression was so menacing, so overpowering that I had to force myself to dwell in her presence. I had to literally sit on my hands so as not to busy myself checking her latest coagulation test results on the computer or scanning the pill bottles for their prescription renewal dates.

She didn't need me to do those mechanical things, at least not at the start of our visit. She needed me to bear witness to her despair. Although there was another doctor responsible for treating her depression, I had to acknowledge the reality of her life – its painful and suffusing darkness. I knew from a previous visit that she had recently been to Latin America for the funeral of her mother. I learned on this visit that a young cousin had just died of the complications of diabetes, raising great fears in the patient that she, too, had diabetes. As a corollary, I discovered that fears of illness, realistic and not, added tremendously to the patient's burden of depression . . .

. . . In retrospect, as I collected myself in private in preparation for the next patient, I realized with a great sense of satisfaction that I had not abandoned her, however strong had been the temptation to do so. I had found a way to be with her – despite not speaking her language and despite my own experiences with depression that she forced me, briefly, to relive – so as to fulfil the duties I incurred by virtue of having heard her [. . .]. The satisfaction I felt was the satisfaction of an internist – not of an ethicist

> *and not of a narratologist, although I am those things too – in my having found a way, today anyway, to be her doctor.'*
>
> (Charon, 2004)

In this example, Charon's evident narrative competence does not remove her obligation to check the dose of the patient's anticoagulants against the evidence-based algorithm, or to make logical choices about how to investigate and manage her back pain, or to do the correct blood test to exclude the much-feared diagnosis of diabetes. Indeed, in her chapter, Charon comments that these 'technical' tasks were much easier to explain and initiate once the more difficult challenge of achieving a common frame for addressing these problems had been accomplished. There was no zero-sum relationship between 'narrative-based' and 'evidence-based' medicine (more of one necessarily requiring less of the other). Rather, as I have argued previously, the former was a prerequisite for the efficient and effective practice of the latter (Greenhalgh, 1999).

In summary, the notion of the 'narrative-based' clinical relationship must go beyond the rather obvious statement that doctors should listen to their patients and not keep interrupting them. The illness narrative is a dialogue, not a monologue, and therein lies its transformative potential. The patient constructs a more coherent, illuminative, hopeful and courageous narrative – and may even create a different self – through their awareness of, and trust in, the perspective of the clinician who is privileged to hear their story.

As illness in general becomes more complex, more multifaceted and more long-term, so narrative competence becomes more critical to the practice of medicine. A working definition of a narrative-competent approach to illness might be that:

- it views the illness, and the patient's efforts to deal with it, as an unfolding story within his or her wider life-world
- it acknowledges the patient as the narrator of the story and as the subject (rather than the object) of the tale, and hence gives central importance to the patient's own role in defining, managing and making sense of the illness
- it recognises that a single problem or experience will generate multiple interpretations, and that the key version to be addressed is the one framed and developed by the patient

- it embraces both trust (the patient makes herself vulnerable and stakes confidence in the clinician in the act of telling her story) and obligation (the clinician incurs ethical duties in the act of hearing it)
- it views the spoken (and enacted) dialogue between health professional and patient as an integral part of the clinical management.

But as I hope I have demonstrated by the worked examples in this chapter, narrative competence does not absolve the clinician of the duty to base his or her recommendations on the best available scientific evidence. Indeed, I believe passionately that the narrative-competent clinician will be better able to draw appropriately and judiciously on the tools and techniques of evidence-based medicine, to apply sensitivity and common sense to the application of evidence to this particular case, and to communicate the 'evidence' to the patient in a way that is personally relevant and culturally congruent.

Chapter Three

Stories and learning

The story of Mrs Uddin

Mrs Uddin is a 35-year-old Bengali woman. She is 20 weeks pregnant and already has three children. Mrs Uddin recently came to this country and was diagnosed with diabetes. She had to face many difficulties. She was missing her family in Bangladesh. Her husband works outside London and visits twice a week. She therefore stays with her in-laws. Mrs Uddin was expecting her husband to take her to the GP. She was feeling very tired. When she eventually saw the midwife she found out that she was diabetic. She had to start taking insulin, for which she was dependent on others. Her grandmother and father had also been diabetic. Her father had not taken care of his health and he died at age 50.

Learning she was insulin dependent was frightening for Mrs Uddin and caused her to become depressed. She did not understand why she had to take insulin and thought it might cause her to die like her father. Due to language barriers that existed, Mrs Uddin found it difficult to get the necessary help when she needed it. She relied on her sister-in-law to inject her with insulin, but she often had to wait long times for her medication as her sister-in-law was busy. Mrs Uddin had been to the hospital a few times. The link worker and health advocate had been regularly monitoring her progress and feeding back the information to the health professionals.

Why did you choose this story?

Because of the many difficulties Mrs Uddin had to face being diagnosed with diabetes away from home.

What questions or issues does this story raise?

Through the advocates Mrs Uddin realised that not taking her insulin properly would result in detrimental effects on her unborn baby.

What are the learning points?

Mrs Uddin became much more responsible for her own health and had more help from her extended family once they had gained knowledge about the condition and how to treat it. Mrs Uddin did not previously understand diabetes and found it difficult to treat herself. After being advised by the link worker and health advocate, Mrs Uddin realised the seriousness of her condition and sorted out taking her medication regularly.

Tutor's comment

This story illustrates a number of themes commonly found in a family with diabetes. First, there is a positive family history and a 'horror story' of a relative with early death. Second, the family members with previous experience of caring for diabetes are not the ones who are around when a new case is diagnosed (in this case, because they are back in Bangladesh). Third, contrary to the popular stereotype, the support from this Asian extended family is inadequate – those who are competent to help also have their own lives to lead. Finally, there is a strong suggestion of both guilt and despair in the diabetic member: she is dependent on her relatives but also conscious of being a burden to them.

Reproduced with permission from the *Sharing Stories Workbook* (Greenhalgh & Collard, 2003)

The story, written up as homework on a 'sharing stories' course for bilingual health advocates,[6] was first told orally in a small group of three within a larger seminar of about 15 participants. The format of the seminar, as the name suggests, was one of informal story-sharing. The theme that the group had asked to cover that week was 'diabetes in the family' (interestingly, this double meaning was reflected in the content of the stories, which covered both the hereditary nature of diabetes and the role of the family in supporting the diabetic member). The task that I had set the group was to 'share some stories about your clients with diabetes and their families'. After 15 minutes or so in which each group of three chatted quietly among themselves, I invited them to offer their 'best stories' for the wider seminar group to comment on.

The atmosphere when the advocates were discussing in small groups

[6] Bilingual health advocates are more than medical interpreters. As well as translating in clinical consultations, they work as support workers and 'cultural brokers' for people from minority ethnic groups, some of whom struggle against multiple disadvantage (poverty, poor housing, inadequate access to services, and chronic illness – as well as the obvious difficulty of a language barrier) (Angelelli, 2005).

was very relaxed, because sharing a story between two or three people is almost always an informal act. There was often silence initially as participants tried to think of stories that fitted the agreed theme. Occasionally, one person was very keen to share a story – perhaps because it was especially memorable or tragic, but more often because it had happened very recently (maybe the same morning), or because an aspect of the problem was still pressing. The listeners did what listeners do – they heard the account, asked questions, and reacted appropriately to the literary tropes used – with amusement, shock, disbelief, empathy, or just nods of understanding. Sometimes they offered similar or contrasting stories on the same theme.

In these sessions we never formally defined what a 'good story' was (*see* page 9), but the best stories were easy to spot from my position in a corner of the room, because the small group in which that story was being shared would become especially animated. They would make more noise, and there would be giggles, groans, or even screams. This small group might announce to the wider group 'We've got a good one', and wait impatiently for the time I called them all together to hear the best stories. Sometimes individuals in one group would be distracted into listening to the 'good story' in an adjacent group instead of concentrating on the less interesting tale being told in their own group.

When I announced that it was time to hear the 'good stories', everyone knew where to look – and without fail a story with many potential learning points would emerge (often as a re-telling by someone who had been a listener in their own small group, but now sought the narrator role). We would discuss the learning points not within a formal, pre-set syllabus but as questions arising from the story.

Why did Mrs Uddin think that the insulin was going to harm her? This question drew half a dozen or so similar narratives about the advocates' Bangladeshi clients who had negative perceptions about insulin. People with diabetes can be fine for years, but when they get put on insulin, it's often only a year or two before they die – or so the stories suggested. To place this in perspective, I had to put on my medical hat and explain that the natural course of type 2 diabetes is to get steadily worse with time. The commonly seen progression from dietary treatment to tablets to insulin followed this illness trajectory, and hence the need for insulin was often a symptom, not a cause, of life-threatening deterioration. More stories were offered to support – and to challenge – my explanation, and I was required to introduce more medical detail to explain apparent inconsistencies in the other stories.

Another concern raised by this story was the perception amongst this strictly Muslim group that insulin is taken from dead cows (it isn't, but even some of the advocates didn't know this). In a group activity later in the seminar series, mainly as a result of the stories sparked by this index case, the advocates designed a patient information leaflet about insulin. It had as its first line, in capital letters, 'THIS DOES NOT COME FROM A COW'. We learned from real stories that some Bangladeshi clients would read (or listen) no further if they had not been reassured of this fact at the outset.

When I later compared this leaflet with the official advice leaflet in Bengali (translated pretty much word for word from its English equivalent), there was around 50% homology. In other words, half the information provided in the English leaflet never featured in the stories told about Bangladeshi clients, and half the genuine information needs of Bangladeshis identified from the advocates' stories were not met by the topics covered in the English leaflet. Neither leaflet was scientifically incorrect, but only one began 'THIS DOES NOT COME FROM A COW'.

Why didn't Mrs Uddin's sister-in-law organise herself to give her the insulin injections on a more regular basis? Why should she? This question drew a heated discussion about the expectations placed on 'Asian' women to provide an extended carer role, unpaid and untrained. Surely the real issue here was not the sister-in-law's failure to provide 24-hour care, but the inaccessibility of the NHS system to a frightened and socially isolated woman with limited English proficiency? The group was not agreed on this. We heard counter-narratives about Bangladeshi families who cared much better and more willingly for their diabetic relative than the woman in the index story. We explored cultural, religious and gender aspects of the traditional Asian carer role and talked about how it had become more difficult as lifestyles (especially those of women) had become more 'westernised'. We learned that there is no right answer to questions about what 'should' happen in families, and most participants agreed with the suggestion that, as professionals, our role is to respond appropriately to what *does* happen rather than to impose our personal view of what *should* happen. Some of the less experienced advocates found this difficult to grasp initially, and persisted in offering rather dogmatic statements about what is and isn't expected of a good sister-in-law or a good Muslim. They went home still pondering about the nature of professionalism, and brought more stories on this theme the following week.

I've told you this story about my advocates' story-sharing group because it illustrates a number of general points about the use of stories in teaching and learning. But before we consider the theoretical aspects of storytelling in learning, we need to understand the nature of learning itself. Adult (or experiential) learning theory goes back over 50 years to the work of child psychologist Jean Piaget, sociologist Kurt Lewin and educationist John Dewey (Kolb, 1993). The experiential learning cycle (*see* Figure 3.1) emphasises the role of active experience and reflection in shaping understanding (Kolb, 1993). Lewin believed that the failure to learn effectively was usually attributable to a lack of adequate feedback to feed the process of reflection, resulting in an imbalance between observation and action.

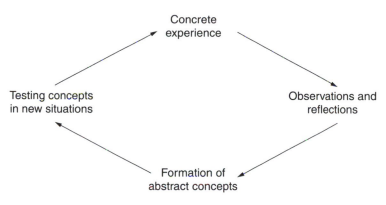

Figure 3.1 The experiential learning cycle (Lewin and Kolb).

Dewey's model of experiential learning is similar to that of Lewin, but places more emphasis on *ideas* as an impetus for learning (Kolb, 1993). Dewey depicts a progressive spiral in which judgements based on concrete observations lead the learner, via new ideas, closer to an ultimate purpose or goal (*see* Figure 3.2). These and other experiential learning theories differ fundamentally from both instructivist theories (which depict learning in terms of the accumulation of facts, like storing money in a bank, and which assume that learning can be assessed by the reproduction of these facts) and behaviourist theories (which depict learning in terms of performance outputs, like teaching a dog to beg for a reward, and which deny – or at least refuse to analyse – any key role of meaning making in the learning process).

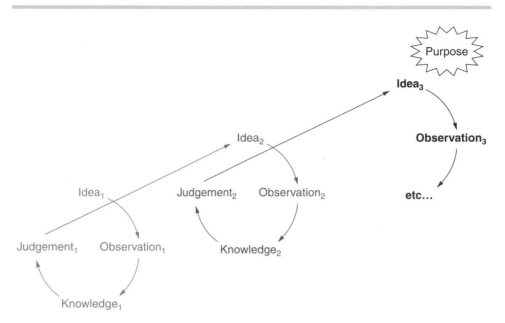

Figure 3.2 Dewey's purpose-oriented, developmental learning spiral.

Experiential learning theories assume that facts are not fixed and immutable elements of thought but are constantly formed and re-formed through reflection, experience and feedback. Such approaches view learning as a continuous process in which every new experience builds on, and integrates with, the accumulated experiences that have gone before. Thus, says Kolb, no two thoughts are ever the same, since experience always intervenes (Kolb, 1993). Most importantly for the focus of this chapter, experiential learning theories give central importance to social discourse as a means of promoting reflection and consolidating or changing understanding. As Paulo Friere put it, *'Knowledge emerges only through invention and reinvention, through the restless, impatient, continuing, hopeful inquiry men pursue in the world, with the world, and with each other'* (Friere, 1974).

As my example of the advocates' workshop showed, the story is a powerful trigger for Friere's 'restless, impatient, continuing, hopeful inquiry'. A story told twice is a different story, and any narrative shared in a group draws both supporting narratives (which follow similar plots and hence construe actions, events and their causes and consequences similarly) and counter-narratives (which by definition pursue different plots, thereby construing the 'same' action or event in an alternative causal sequence). The story is not only holistic (that is, it covers all aspects of experience and the context in which that experience must be interpreted) but also incompressible (that is, it cannot be summarised without losing meaning). Because the story is a personal construal of what led to what, and of why so-and-so did X, it conveys the narrator's unique and perspectival understanding of the world. It also conveys that person's construction of how the main characters in the story in turn construe the world.

All this is rich material for experiential learning. The adult learning cycle (*see* Figure 3.1) or spiral (*see* Figure 3.2) does not progress by individual accumulation of new facts and experiences, but by the construction of these facts and experiences into meaningful stories and the sharing of these stories with critical others. In a learning group – either formally established (as in a learning set) or informally gathered (as in a coffee queue at a conference or around a family dinner table) – learners' stories are the vehicle through which the meaning of a shared or common experience is negotiated and reframed. Stories are placed by members of the learning group into a rummage-bin of ideas, experiences and observations that can be drawn upon in discussion.

If you have ever used stories in teaching, you will know that even the dullest group of learners perks up when a story is told. The story is a natural and universal form of communication – we all learned how to listen to stories at our mother's knee. Stories are inherently engaging because they are image-rich, action-packed, laden with emotions and suffused with meaning. Because they are explicitly subjective and perspectival, stories invite the ongoing negotiation of meaning between teller and listener. The story is the narrator's, but it is inherently dialogic (*see* my discussion of Bakhtin's notion of 'otherness' on page 21). It is entirely socially acceptable for a listener to challenge the causal relationships implicit in a storyteller's emplotment of events (as enacted, for example, in the pantomime audience's refrain, 'Oh no it isn't'). And stories reflect the complexity of real life by their holistic and multifaceted nature. In a story, as in real life, 'diabetes in the family' is both about the genetics of diabetes inheritance *and* about the role of the family in the practical and social support of the diabetic member.

Stories offer insights into what *might* (or *could* or *should*) have been, and hence offer the opportunity (indeed, the implicit requirement) to consider different options and their likely endings. This is what Bruner has called subjunctivisation – and it is a property of stories that is especially useful in teaching and learning (Bruner, 1990). Asking the class to 'give the story a different ending' can be a fast track to identifying what have been called PUNs (patients' unmet needs) and DENs (doctors' and other professionals' educational needs) (Eve, 2003). 'If only I had known about the guideline, I might have spared Mrs X an operation' is an example of the learning potential of subjunctivisation inherent in the storying of problems. In addition, as I discuss in Chapter Six (Stories and ethics), stories have an important ethical dimension, and hence can serve as powerful motivators for the learner (Rubin, 2002).

Stories told in professional groups are very often about professional identity. Sharing stories about 'diabetes in the family' prompts multiple constructions of what it is to be an advocate trying to help someone with diabetes to make sense of their illness, promote appropriate support from their family, and take action to reduce the risk of children inheriting the condition. Multiple shared stories on the same topic convey the diversity of professional experience – but they also highlight common themes raised by clients (specific information needs, folk models of illness, fears), common aspects of context (poverty, comorbidity, religious constraints), ethical dilemmas (such as poor performance or racism in healthcare staff), and tensions in professional roles ('impartial translator' versus 'cultural broker'). Intra-group discussion about what a particular story *means* fuels the learning cycle, especially if skilled facilitation prompts the group to seek knowledge from external sources (experts, books or databases) at the critical point in the cycle.

Another theoretical advantage of the story form in teaching and learning, which I mentioned briefly in Chapter One, is what Aristotle called universality (Aristotle, 1996b). Every story is unique, yet it is also generalisable – because story is not about what *did* happen in a strictly historical sense, but about what *could* happen. A child with insulin-dependent diabetes used his friend's needle because he forgot his own. From a learning perspective, we don't much care if the child in the story really did use his friend's needle, because the story rings true as one that could happen, given what we know about the forgetfulness of young boys, the camaraderie and reciprocity between friends who have diabetes, and public ignorance about blood-borne infections. Similarly, the actual level of helpfulness of Mrs Uddin's sister-in-law (*see* page 33) is of less educational significance than the general narrative truth that the story conveys (i.e. that not all members of Asian extended families conform to the popular stereotype held by health professionals).

On occasion, the story's implicit claim to universality is entirely unjustified – as in the apocryphal individual who smoked heavily and lived to 95, or the unfortunate diabetic person who went blind and had both legs amputated before reaching the age of 40. This produces a hypothetical danger that people in informal story-sharing groups might share 'wrong' stories, thus leading each other astray. But these fears are, I think, built on a naive model of learning – that the learner accumulates 'facts' (including incorrect ones), which lead directly to a change in behaviour. As I explained on page 37, contemporary theories of adult learning suggest that it is a much more fluid and complex process, based on active and collaborative efforts at sense making. Unless 'wrong' stories are entirely outside the experience of other members of the learning group (and often even if they are), they invariably draw passionate counter-narratives and an active search for further knowledge to resolve the issue. Indeed, some of the most dynamic and effective learning sessions I have experienced both as a learner and as a teacher have been triggered by just such a 'wrong story.'

The crucial role of the facilitator of the learning group is to capture these tensions around 'wrong stories' and turn them into learning opportunities, for example, by encouraging the group members to seek independent evidence to adjudicate between the truth-value of different stories, or to invite experts along who will adjudicate on their behalf. This is the difference between an effective learning group and a dysfunctional one. In the past, I have attended lay support groups in which the only stories shared seem to be apocalyptic tales told (and ritually re-told) by die-hard group members with unusually serious complications of the condition or unusually unlucky brushes with the system. Such groups tend to be characterised not just by lack of an identifiable facilitator, but also by a more general lack of reflection and by the inability of many group members to get a word in edgeways. The difference between this sort of story-sharing group and one that is competently facilitated cannot be over-emphasised – but as I shall argue in the next section, the role of the facilitator is emphatically not to move into didactic mode whenever there is tension within the group.

Anthropologist Dr Anna Collard and I wrote many grant applications to try to extend the 'sharing stories' learning groups from bilingual health advocates to people with diabetes, whom we believed had as much to learn from stories as healthcare professionals. Our previous research had shown that positive lifestyle changes (such as giving up smoking) in British Bangladeshis are almost always attributed by them to a story told in an informal setting by another Bangladeshi (Greenhalgh *et al.*, 1998). Despite this, funding bodies were initially reluctant to provide financial support for something as informal, subjective, unpredictable and plain anecdotal as story-sharing groups.

A common criticism of our plans (indeed, the most usual reason given for turning us down), to which I alluded above, was the risk that 'wrong stories' would be shared. Another concern was that patients would talk about trivial matters and might not cover the most crucial aspects of the diabetes 'syllabus'. The implicit assumption in the rejection letters was that a more rigorous and scientific approach to teaching patients about diabetes would be for professionals to set the agenda and stick to a structured, standardised and 'evidence-based' curriculum (Cavan & Cradock, 2004). This, of course, is only true if you take an instructivist perspective on learning (learning being the 'filling of a bucket' with items of knowledge). If you take an experiential perspective, there can be no such thing as a 'standardised' curriculum in the strict sense, since every learner has a different set of prior experiences and personal goals into which new knowledge must be integrated.

We did eventually secure funding to extend our story-sharing groups to people with diabetes, and we established several such groups in community centres and lunch clubs.[7] The storytelling took a very different format from the advocates' workshops (in which we had been able to organise the group and invite storytelling and reflection in a structured and timetabled way). The people with diabetes (who were mostly Sylheti- or Gujarati-speaking immigrants with little or no English), in contrast, were not willing to sit around in a circle taking turns telling stories, nor were they willing to be organised or facilitated by the research team. Discussion generally took the form of animated arguments between participants, which Anna and I were called in periodically to resolve. Multiple conversations could often be heard simultaneously, and participants wandered about the room, coming and going as they pleased and sometimes bringing friends or grand-children with them.

One important finding from our observation of the diabetes groups was the strong action orientation. Doing took precedence over talking. For example, many women attended the group to check their blood glucose levels on our meter, even though we had provided them with their own

[7] We received funding from Diabetes UK for action research on the story-sharing groups. The initial research that identified 'a story told by another Bangladeshi' as critical to health-related action was funded by the Wellcome Trust. We are grateful to all these funders, and to the participants in the groups, for taking the risk of supporting this unconventional approach to diabetes education.

meters and shown them how to use them. In one group, a woman who had had a needle phobia for years initially shied away from the meter, but after seeing her colleagues queue to test their blood on arrival week on week, she eventually disclosed a strong desire to overcome her aversion to testing. It took several sessions for her to agree to have her finger pricked (to much cheering and applause). Within a few more weeks, this woman had taken over the use of the meter and tested everyone on arrival, taking personal responsibility for talking round any newcomer who was reluctant to be tested.

In another group, at which the agreed topic of discussion was medication, a woman produced a large carrier bag of tablets, including several boxes of the anti-diabetic drug metformin, whose known side-effects include abdominal pain and excessive wind. This prompted similar stories by several others about the 'big white pills', and one participant physically enacted being stuck on the toilet groaning while a grandchild was calling for her attention from the living room. There was much discussion about the hospital doctor's refusal to take these side-effects sufficiently seriously to offer a change in medication. Small wonder then that most of the boxes of metformin were unopened.

The mechanism by which sharing stories in groups improves the illness experience of someone with diabetes is still speculative (and is a focus of some continuing research by my own team[8]). Group education in diabetes produces better biomedical outcomes than individual education, even when stories are not explicitly used as the vehicle for learning (Trento *et al.*, 2002; Koev *et al.*, 2003). The mechanisms by which such groups achieve an effect on members' learning might include the following:

- an enhanced learning environment – because multiple opportunities often exist to learn visually, aurally and by doing (Elwyn *et al.*, 2000)
- the development of self-efficacy, defined by social psychologist Albert Bandura as *'the belief in one's ability to organise and execute the courses of action required to manage prospective situations'* (Bandura, 1995). Knowledge of facts will not lead to change in behaviour if the individual lacks confidence and/or the belief that their actions will make a real difference. Bandura (among others) has shown that self-efficacy is

---

[8] We are currently comparing the 'sharing stories' approach to diabetes education with conventional approaches in a randomised controlled trial. This trial commenced in early 2006 and is funded by the UK Department of Health Service Delivery and Organisation Programme. See www.newhamuniversityhospital.co.uk/poseidon/

built through supervised practical exercises in which the learner receives feedback on the success of their efforts[9]

- development of social capital such as friends, contacts and local knowledge (Wenger, 1996; Schuller *et al.*, 2004).

The use of members' own stories in a group learning session adds to the potential mechanisms for learning – by, for example:

- social learning (learning by modelling). This is another term introduced by Bandura. In his words, *'Of the many cues that influence behaviour, at any point in time, none is more common than the actions of others'* (Bandura, 1986). The story serves to put into words, or indeed to enact directly, the behaviour that forms the 'lesson'. The key mechanism of social learning is vicarious experience – that is, being inspired to action (or put off) by what happened to someone else, as illustrated by our 'needle phobia' lady on page 43, who for many others with a similar problem became a living example of how to overcome this handicap
- transmission and personalisation of 'tacit' knowledge – that is, practical know-how that is difficult to articulate formally and which isn't often found in books or leaflets (Polanyi, 1962; Eraut, 1999). When a group member says that she would like to cook 'healthy' curries but her husband does not find them tasty, she will generally be met with a deluge of advice on making healthy curries tasty using particular cooking methods and spices from the local shop
- collective sense making – in which the group questions, reflects on, negotiates and reframes the meaning of information until it is expressed in a way that is acceptable, meaningful and sensible (Weick, 1995). Stories, especially those told orally in a group, are sense-making devices because they allow events to be ordered and interpreted, and then re-ordered and re-interpreted so that different meanings and motives can be considered
- reframing of identity – for example, reconstructing the self from 'victim

[9] Self-efficacy is a popular theme in contemporary UK health education policy because it forms the cornerstone of self-management of chronic illness in the Department of Health's Expert Patient Programme (Department of Health, 2001). Lay-led training programmes in self-management are currently advocated for a number of chronic illnesses (Bury *et al.*, 2005). Such programmes differ from the story-sharing approach described in this chapter in that there is a predefined syllabus which the lay educators are expected to cover, and the personal story, while not explicitly discouraged, is not seen to have any special educational significance. I have argued in this chapter that the story-sharing approach has a number of theoretical advantages over didactic health education or lay-led syllabus-driven programmes, but these advantages have yet to be demonstrated empirically.

of my diabetes' to 'on top of my diabetes', or from 'passive accepter of my doctor's advice' to 'active challenger of my doctor's advice' (Goffman, 1969)
* 'healing drama' – that is, the enacting of a positive personal story (Mattingly, 1998).

This last mechanism in particular is worth exploring further. The performative nature of the stories in our patient support groups (*see* page 43), in which drama rather than talk was the basis of communication, was probably the most important finding of this phase of our research. In an evaluation session about a year after the group began, we asked the members of one of the story-sharing groups what they would tell a friend about the group. One very perceptive comment was that '*If someone has diabetes and doesn't know what to do, they should come to the group first, and they will learn what to do*'.

The powerful potential of group story-sharing to link illness narrative with practical action accords particularly well with Aristotle's definition of tragedy as '*an imitation of an action that is serious, complete, and of a certain magnitude; in language embellished with artistic ornament, the several kinds being found in separate parts of the play; in the form of action, not of [spoken or written] narrative; with incidents arousing pity and fear, wherewith to accomplish catharsis of the emotions*' (Aristotle, 1996b).

This famous definition, originally written in relation to a scholarly analysis of theatre in ancient Greece, needs more interpretation if we seek to apply it to patient education in the twenty-first century. My own reading of Aristotle suggests three key principles which we can apply to the example of the woman whose clinic doctor persisted in prescribing a drug that had given her intolerable abdominal upset (*see* page 43). First, tragedy (one of several possible narrative plots, as described on page 6) works particularly well as a performance, and hence an illness narrative with a tragic twist acquires special poignance when enacted amongst a sympathetic audience. Second, the arousal of emotion in the audience can be cathartic for the actor – the audience's expression of pity and fear (and presumably other emotions such as horror or indignation) can prove empowering for the person whose illness narrative forms the focus of the drama. Third, a good tragedy is balanced and complete, so the enactment of an unfinished illness narrative generates a certain ethical obligation within the group to help the individual to set the tragic events straight (or, if that is not possible, to see the story through to its inevitable ending). This audience did not merely acknowledge the 'stuck on the toilet' narrative as an unreasonable situation for our heroine to be put in. Through their response (anger, outrage, empathy) to the enactment of the story, they became a source of indignant affirmation that the woman should return for a stand-off with the junior doctor about changing the medication.

I have argued elsewhere that storytelling is not a panacea for effective teaching or learning (Greenhalgh, 2001). As Mrs Uddin's story on page 33 illustrates, stories are useful for 'living through' the perspective of people whose illness experience is vastly different from our own (religious or ethnic minorities, the very old, the very sick, or someone of a different gender). Because the story is about human action in the face of trouble, because it embraces complexity, and because it raises possibilities, stories are also especially powerful in considering 'what to do' in complex practical situations where there is an ethical dimension. As the examples in this chapter have shown, this makes them especially useful in developing professional practice and in supporting what is popularly known as 'self-management' of chronic illness (*see* footnote, page 44).

In summary, stories are powerful tools for teaching and learning. Despite folk models and media images to the contrary, both the experience of illness and the practice of healthcare are complex and highly subjective affairs, shot through with ambiguity and with clinical and ethical uncertainty. For both healthcare professionals seeking to provide effective care and patients seeking to develop mastery of their own illness, learning 'what to do' in particular situations is often more critical to success than accumulating decontextualised 'facts'. The inherent characteristics of the story form – image-rich, action-oriented, emplotted, complex, malleable, dynamic, negotiable, and alluding to what could be or what might have been – make it uniquely suited to the support of experiential learning either formally (as in a learning set) or informally wherever learners meet to make sense of the material they have covered.

There is much we don't yet know about how best to use stories in teaching and learning, and with regard to robust research evidence on what works best for whom, and in what circumstances, the main message is still 'watch this space'. If you are seeking a practical guide to using stories in professional education, I recommend Janice McDrury and Maxine Alterio's book *Learning Through Storytelling in Higher Education* (McDrury & Alterio, 2002), and also the workbook that Anna Collard and I wrote for the advocates on our 'sharing stories' project (Greenhalgh & Collard, 2003).

Chapter Four

Stories and organisations

My family and I always believed that the NHS provided the best treatment in the world. We now know that this is not the case. David, my father, died late last night in your hospital after his long fight against cancer. He was admitted three days ago to be operated on to alleviate his symptoms. He was starved for 24 hours in readiness for the operation. The operation was cancelled on the first day and then again the day after that. You simply cannot starve cancer patients for days on end in the hope that their operation might be carried out. Is this any way to treat a person in the last three days of their life on this earth? I am shocked and amazed that you consider the management of my father's case and the administration of his treatment to be of a good standard.

Comment in a Visitors' Book in a hospital chapel. Reproduced with permission from 'The role of stories and storytelling in organisational change efforts' (Bate, 2004).

Narrative approaches seek to understand organisations, and also drive change, via the stories told within them and the stories told about them. In the previous chapter, I suggested that the story has a number of advantages as a tool for learning. Many of these same characteristics make stories a uniquely useful tool for understanding and attempting to change organisations.

The first of these advantages is that stories embrace complexity and are embedded in other stories. Organisations are complex entities with fuzzy and inconstant boundaries. What we call 'the organisation' means different things to different people, and it changes from day to day and year to year. Large public-sector healthcare organisations are more complex than most, and those in the UK are embedded in the wider National Health Service, itself part of the Welfare State, and linked (to a greater or lesser extent in any locality) with social services, schools, the voluntary sector, and so on. Even something as superficially simple as a GP surgery or a hospital clinic is remarkably difficult to draw out on the back of an envelope – which is why stories about the NHS are often so much more meaningful than the charts and flow diagrams that are supposed to represent its structure and lines of accountability. Events in any story unfold because of the dynamic interplay of the actions of different players, each of whom is variously enabled and constrained by the context(s) in which the action happens. Thus storytelling, although conventionally seen as an untidy, meandering and needlessly discursive means of representing reality, may actually be the clearest and most efficient means of capturing the organisational dimension of the illness experience or the provision of healthcare.

One technique that we all use unconsciously to convey and make sense of complexity is what Boje has called 'terse stories'. Stories in organisations rarely come fully formed with a beginning, middle and end linked by a plot. More often, people speak in story fragments – that is, brief accounts that are not in themselves coherent or meaningful, but which make sense when placed in the wider cultural and historical context and mental schemata shared by the organisation's members (Boje, 1991). For example, the statement 'the boss is late again' told informally in an organisation draws on a shared understanding among the staff of the boss's previous behaviour, the meaning the staff attach to that behaviour, and their assumptions (true or not) about the boss's personality and private life. The essence of a terse story is not what is stated in the fragment but what remains *unstated*, since these are the elements that do not need to be expressed. These unstated elements are the researcher's clues to the shared assumptions and perspectives on reality that make up organisational culture – about which more in Chapter Five (Stories and research).

The second advantage of stories in an organisational setting, and one which is especially relevant in relation to organisational change, is their sense-making potential (Weick, 1995). To be successfully assimilated by members of the organisation, a proposed change must make sense in a way that relates to previous understanding and experience. People caught up in a change initiative (or who are trying to 'stay afloat' in a changing environment) engage in a continuous stream of experience and action, which generates a succession of equivocal situations. They then *retrospectively impose* a structure or schema to make these situations sensible. In other words, the act of sense making is itself the construction of a narrative, requiring elements to be selected out, highlighted as significant or surprising, juxtaposed with one another and with existing cognitive schemata, and thereby given meaning. The story serves as both an anchor and a springboard in times of rapid change.

'When a decision is at hand, the old stories are recounted and compared to unfolding story lines to keep the organisation from repeating historically bad

> *choices and to invite the repetition of past successes. In a turbulent environment, the organisational halls and offices pulsate with a story life of the here and now that is richer and more vibrant than the firm's environment.'*
>
> (Boje, 1991)

Some organisational anthropologists have gone so far as to argue that storytelling is essential to adaptation and survival in large, impersonal, bureaucratic and technology-dominated institutions (Czarniawska, 1998; Gabriel, 2000). Imagine learning how to be a doctor, nurse, volunteer or chaplain (or indeed to play any other organisational role) in the NHS without the use of stories. I recently organised a work-experience week for a group of 16-year-old school pupils at my local hospital. The pupils made very little use of the written guidance I had painstakingly produced on what (not) to wear, where (not) to go and what (not) to do. Of far more use to them were the stories told in tea-breaks by my medical-student helpers of incidents when they had been caught eating crisps on a ward round, inadvertently upended a patient's dinner by sitting on a bed, or turned up to Professor So-and-So's teaching session in a risqué T-shirt. These informal stories conveyed the organisational dos and don'ts far more effectively than my structured lists – and they also humanised and personalised organisational culture in a way that the formal instructions had failed to do.

The third characteristic of stories relevant to organisational studies is that they are memorable. Stories are image-rich, action-packed and full of surprises. Just as the story is the unit of individual memory (Hinchman & Hinchman, 1997), the folklore passed on through stories is a key element of institutional memory (Gabriel, 2000). 'Learning the ropes' in an organisation often includes picking up stories about people who left years ago but whose actions or experiences have become woven into stories told by present-day staff and clients. Stories about the much-loved previous chief executive, for example, may set the context for a general lament about the weaknesses of the present incumbent of the post.

Fourth, stories can reveal the counter-culture of an organisation – in which the seeds of change can very often be seen. Funny stories in particular, shared by low-status staff in informal space when the boss is not around, serve to reveal absurdities, assign alternative identities to key characters, expose red tape, and draw attention to inequities such as oppression or disempowerment of staff or patients (Humphreys & Brown,

2002; Stone-Mediatore, 2003). Yiannis Gabriel's fieldwork has highlighted the contrast between organisations' official version of their own story ('well-oiled machine, cutting-edge technology') and the subversive metaphors used by the members ('the [pompous, incompetent] management, nothing works round here') (Gabriel, 2000).

Subversive stories feed the creative imagination of organisational innovators (Buckler & Zein, 1996; Higgins & McAllaster, 2002). They create the backdrop for new visions and embody permission to break the rules. In an old-fashioned machine bureaucracy, behaviours and events that go beyond the existing structures and systems are implicitly (and often explicitly) 'wrong'. Telling a story about someone with a new idea allows their actions to be imbued with meaning and the change agent to be accorded positive qualities such as courage, creativity, and so on ('Mrs Fernando from the records department went in and told the consultant straight, and you should have seen the look on his face').

Fifth, stories are a vital window not only to the truths about the organisation, but also to its fictions – in which, for example, key characters are unjustifiably canonised or demonised in stories that are closer to gossip than to fact. Provided that we keep the status of these fictions in mind, they can reveal aspects of the organisation that are otherwise inaccessible to the student of its culture. Indeed, an important theoretical point to grasp is that organisations cannot be understood via the 'facts' alone. One organisational anthropologist has claimed that *'Modern institutions . . . run on fictions, and the task of the scholar is to study how these fictions are created and sustained'* (Czarniawska, 1998). Through stories, members of an organisation interpret events, infusing them with meaning by linking them in temporal (implicitly causal) sequence, and through distortions, omissions, embellishments, metaphors and other literary devices. Not only is the 'true' version of events an unhelpful concept, but also the very plasticity of stories in organisations is the key to what Gabriel has called the 'organisational dreamworld' (Gabriel, 2000).

Here is an example. I recently attended a seminar in which we discussed several transcripts of interviews with senior executives about the takeover of one large organisation by another. More than one interviewee had referred to the practice of counting the toilet rolls, which had (allegedly) been introduced across the board the day after the merger. In some ways it didn't matter whether the stories were 'true' (did staff members really have to account for every sheet of toilet paper?) or not. It was their choice of metaphor that was significant. The toilet-paper story perfectly symbolised the new culture of the merged organisation. Micro-management extended everywhere, even behind the locked lavatory door (perhaps the ultimate place where decent people might expect to be left in privacy). There was a performance standard for everything, including bodily functions, and staff had been told that they had failed to meet it. It wasn't just that the new management did not trust people who had given decades of faithful service to the old organisation. They were perceived to feel that long-standing senior employees had been spending too much time with their trousers down all those years. This example illustrates how the study of 'fictions' can illuminate some of the most inaccessible issues in organisational life.

One final feature of storytelling that is critical in the organisational context is its links to leadership. Leaders are people who tell good stories, and about whom good stories are told (Gardner, 1995). A good organisational leader is one who can not only develop a vision of where the organisation is heading, but also articulate that vision in terms of an ongoing, enacted story about who we all are and where we are going, thereby *putting the "us" in "me" and the "me" in "us"* (Bate, 2004). Most of us know the feeling of futility and disengagement that occurs when change is imposed by means of executive letters, must-do memos and other devices for conveying top-down instructions through a bureaucracy. Most of us have also experienced the stirring in our hearts when someone we admire and respect gives a speech or writes a letter that voices a vision for change in which we feel personally and actively engaged. Every chief executive, senior partner or clinical director yearns to achieve a fraction of the personal charisma and rhetorical power used by Martin Luther King in *'I have a dream . . .'* or by Churchill in *'We shall fight them on the beaches . . .'*[10] – and it is no accident that both of these famous speeches were composed almost entirely of stories.

In the previous chapter, I used a mainstream theoretical model (experiential learning theory) to illustrate how, and under what conditions, stories might enhance learning by individuals. In order to use stories effectively in organisational change, we must first understand change from a theoretical perspective.[11] In classical management theory, change management is all about defining clear objectives and ensuring that these

[10] Original recordings of both of these famous speeches are easily obtainable as downloads from the Internet if you put the first line into Google.
[11] The organisational change literature is about as theoretically inconsistent as any I have ever encountered. I hope you will forgive me for presenting a very eclectic summary of this complex and contested territory.

happen by (for example) appointing the right staff, providing the right training, making resources available for defined projects, and keeping everyone fixed on clear goals and milestones (Iles & Sutherland, 1998). According to this perspective, change is – at least implicitly – something that can be planned, put on people's job descriptions, managed pro-actively, and audited against predefined success criteria.

But classical management theory has been largely superseded by a number of more contemporary models of organisational change (Bate, 1994). In one such view, change is not a technical process that can (or should) be 'properly managed', but a process dependent on the con-struction, acquisition, transfer and use of knowledge, and on the need for the members of an organisation to make sense of change efforts by assimilating them into their cognitive schemata. Perhaps the best-known writer on knowledge-based views of organisations is Peter Senge, author of *The Learning Organisation* (Senge, 1994). A learning organisation is one in which the acquisition and sharing of knowledge by its members are valued and actively facilitated (for example, through seminars, informal discussions, training days, and appropriate IT infra-structure and support). The notion of organisational change as the reframing and sense making of knowledge by its members aligns with a new conceptualisation of leadership not as 'command and control', but as providing the opportunities and facilitation necessary for people to build and exchange knowledge. In a change effort, the leader's role is to pull a team together around a shared story of innovation, improvement and action. In practice, this means initiating and leading discussions around the *meaning* of any proposed changes.

The quote on page 49 comes from a chapter by Professor Paul Bate, who undertook an action research study to change the culture – and key patient outcomes – in a 'failing' NHS hospital trust. The quote was read out by the chief executive at a multi-professional meeting, and a collective decision to 'do something about this' was subsequently made by those attending. Group members also heard the views of various clinicians, junior and middle managers, and support staff. The group agreed to meet regularly and monitor their efforts to drive the sorts of changes which would ensure that the late David Smith's experience could not occur in the new organisation. Bate's role was to help this happen, and to document progress from both a practical and an academic perspective.

In his chapter, Bate emphasises that change was driven not by himself (the person officially hired as change facilitator) but by the collective social action of the people who had signed up to the change. How did he facilitate this? Mainly, he reflects, by encouraging the group to tell stories, and by offering alternative framings of past or present events and actions, which the other members could choose to run with or reject. In a previous book he has argued about the fundamental role of language in organisational transformation:

> 'If you want to change the way people think, start by changing the way they talk. You need to encourage them to devise new scripts and participate in new language games. You endeavour to shape intellectual and symbolic structures by giving people new topics of conversation to debate, gossip and fight about; and you give them new stories to tell and retell each other. The theory of change is therefore actually quite a simple one: if you can unfreeze and restructure language you can unfreeze and restructure thought . . . Stories and storytelling are a crucial aspect of organisational life . . . the narrative to tie experiences, views and interpretations together, something that has sequence, logic, flow and direction, that represents a coherent version of the emerging reality.'
>
> (Bate, 1994)

If this model of change is taken to its logical conclusion, organisational change is not so much the product of good management as a social movement, embodied in the identities and actions of every member of the organisation. The most readily identifiable social movements are those (such as the feminist movement or the peace movement) that transcend organisations.[12] But change within an organisation can also emerge from the joining together of individual energies. This phenomenon is one that a minority of NHS leaders are now explicitly seeking to capture and exploit at national level – as, for example, in the stirring monograph *Towards a Million Change Agents* (Bate *et al.*, 2005).

> 'Social movements are constituted by the stories people tell to themselves and to one another. They reflect the deepest ways in which people understand who they are and to whom they are connected . . . They are constructed from the interweaving of personal and social biographies – from the narratives people rehearse to themselves about the nature of their lives . . . The construction of

---

[12] For a fascinating account of evidence-based medicine as a social movement, see Cathy Pope's excellent paper (Pope, 2003).

> *collective action, therefore, is inseparable from the construction of personal biography, from the ways, that is, we experience the imprecation of our individual and social selves.'*
>
> (Kling, 1995) (cited in chapter by Bate, 2004)

In his own account of his action research project, and in his general writings on the use of language as a tool in organisational change, Bate presents the development of organisational-level stories as an essentially benign, creative and potentially transforming force that can be captured and channelled by the astute organisational leader or change facilitator. It is worth contrasting this picture with a rather more sinister framing of organisational narrative offered by Rick Iedema and colleagues, who have considered how critical incident reporting (CIR) both reflects and shapes what they call the organisation's 'meta-discourse' (Iedema *et al.*, 2006).

As the airline industry has demonstrated, most disasters arise from human error in imperfect systems. Learning from errors and near misses, and implementing changes (to equipment, staff training, supervision and procedures), are crucial to prevention of similar problems in the future. In CIR, the key staff involved construct a story of what happened, allowing the incident to be analysed at a later date and the findings fed into the quality improvement cycle. The emphasis is not on whose fault the incident was, but on what can be learned from it – and especially the root causes in the system that might be modified (root cause analysis). CIR is generally presented in the literature either as a logico-deductive analytic technique for identifying and correcting flaws in the system, or as a story-based professional learning tool (*see* Chapter Three). Iedema and colleagues propose an alternative perspective – that CIR fundamentally alters the relationship between clinician and organisation through *'the re-articulation of clinical failure into organisational meta-discourse'*. Let me try to explain what they mean by this, because it is relevant to a research technique I'm going to introduce in the next chapter (*see* page 74).

Iedema and colleagues studied CIR in an Australian remote rescue (flying doctor) organisation. They examined 124 written CIR forms (which were structured, interestingly, under four headings – 'Story', 'Outcome', 'Steps taken or treatment required' and 'Was this incident preventable?') using a narrative theoretical lens. In broad terms, they looked for and explored the use of chronology, emplotment, literary devices, emotional comment and dialogic expression (i.e. the extent to which the reporter had implicated a Bakhtinian audience in the narrative, as explained in Chapter Two, page 21). A small proportion of CIR reports seemed explicitly to reject the narrative form by (for example) using telegraphic structure instead of full sentences, lists instead of chronology, passive instead of active voice, and nominalisation rather than verbs (for example, 'demise' rather than 'died'). They found that such a format depersonalised the incident and framed the analysis as a technical study of flaws in system components. But much more commonly, the author used narrative techniques to a greater or lesser extent. In particular, the reports became vivid (and often very moving) stories through the use of chronology, the active voice, dialogism (for example, 'Should I have put a line up at that point?') and insertion of evaluative comments, including personal affect ('I felt angry'), judgements about people ('local doctor had refused to attend') and assessment of contextual factors ('very long distances were involved').

In some examples, narrativising the report appeared to lead successfully to a holistic, no-blame analysis of the problem and the identification of areas for improvement. But in other examples, the more the CIR approximated to the narrative form, the less 'root cause analysis' could be tracked back purely to aspects of the system that could be tweaked. Rather, it exposed interpersonal, inter-professional and inter-organisational tensions that had no easy or universally acceptable solution. In the authors' words, *'narrative confession and mutual scrutiny amongst clinicians need not always produce encouraging outcomes and may give rise to suspicion, resentment and contestation'* (Iedema *et al.*, 2006).

The study described above was undertaken in a particular social and historical context – of increased public and professional awareness of risk and harm in medical care, a rapidly growing culture of managerialism (and the expectation that clinicians should become involved in management), and the increasingly explicit links between the ethical behaviour of doctors and the organisation and management of healthcare (for example, in clinical governance). Applying Foucault's notion of governmentality (i.e. the internalisation and enactment of constraints of state and system by professionals) (Foucault, 1973), the authors argue that the expectation of narrativising of errors in the CIR format puts pressure on doctors to merge their own professional and ethical reflections with organisational norms and expectations, thus blurring the boundary between private and public, individual and state, and clinician and manager. What used to be discussed in confidence (and often informally and 'off the record') between doctors is now a compulsory confessional, recorded in structured CIR format and systematically scrutinised by inter-professional teams through a lens of norms, values, power structures and precedents developed at organisational level (this is what Iedema and colleagues have termed 'organisational meta-discourse').

Iedema and colleagues describe the current era of organisational development as 'post-bureaucracy'. Healthcare organisations have gone beyond the impersonal roles and lines of accountability depicted on the traditional organisational chart,[13] and – as illustrated by the 'confessional' critical incident report – have entered a period in which staff are expected to achieve a deeper level of interrelating and communicating than that explicitly called for on their job description. Whether this is a good thing or not is likely to depend on the particularities of the case and the context. I shall return to this example in the next chapter (*see* page 74), when I use it as an example of a research technique called discourse analysis.

You may or may not agree with Paul Bate that a change facilitator can drive transformation in an organisation by inviting its members to tell different stories to one another, or with Rick Iedema's reframing of critical incident reporting as encroachment of the state and system upon professional identity and practice. But both of these examples should illustrate how a narrative perspective can help us to look at the healthcare organisation in a new light. Through a narrative lens, the organisation moves beyond its traditional image – it ceases to be a machine in which we are all cogs – and becomes (in the first example) a collection of what Charles Handy might call 'resourceful humans' (Handy, 1993) engaged in what Victor Turner would call an unfolding social drama (Turner, 1980), or (in the second example) an overarching set of power relationships and expectations that all of its members internalise, are shaped and constrained by, and – unwittingly and unconsciously – help to perpetuate (Foucault, 1973).

[13] 'Bureaucracy' in the sociological sense has a different meaning from the use of the word to mean unnecessary paperwork. Sociologist Max Weber distinguished between traditional societies, in which a person's status and social role were defined almost exclusively through kinship networks, and modern societies, in which certain roles (in the workplace, for example) are based on the principle that everyone should be treated equally and all have equal responsibilities. In a bureaucratic organisation a person is appointed to a job not because of whose brother-in-law he is but because he has the personal qualities and skills that match the job description (Weber, 1947). Some organisations these days are 'post-bureaucratic' not because they are freed from paperwork (if only!), but because the organisation wants a piece of our soul.

It is a shame, then, that narrative approaches to organisational studies are currently seen as marginal rather than central in the prevailing political climate – which might be summed up in the New Labour slogan 'what matters is what works'. The 'make it happen' mindset of the new public management requires the setting of explicit performance outputs, and depressingly often restricts the focus of both 'quality assurance' and 'research' to establishing the efficiency and cost-effectiveness with which these predefined outputs are achieved (Hammersley, 2001; Webb, 2001). The unpredictable nature of stories, their refusal to be standardised and their tendency to trigger the creative imagination of tellers and listeners make them slippery and frustrating tools when organisational success is defined in such terms. In general, top-down, centralised and managerially driven approaches to organisational change seek to minimise the use of stories and replace them with something more explicit, controllable and auditable (such as an algorithm, protocol or guideline). In the next section I shall describe an example of this tendency which, more than a year after the event, still keeps me awake at night.

The UK Department of Health funds two National Confidential Enquiries every year – into maternal and child health (deaths during pregnancy and in young babies)[14] and into patient outcome and death (serious complications from surgical operations).[15] All health regions are required to submit detailed case reports of any such deaths, and the reasons for the deaths are considered in strict confidence by a multi-professional panel. Traditionally, these reports have been illustrated by case vignettes – stories told by doctors and nurses about the people who died, written in traditional medical jargon and style (*'A 29-year-old primigravida was admitted in the second stage of labour, complaining of a feeling of dizziness . . .'*, etc.). In 2003, the National Institute for Clinical Excellence (NICE) took over responsibility for the Confidential Enquiries (which hitherto had run themselves as quasi-autonomous professional groupings). In 2004, as part of a wider drive towards a more 'evidence-based' approach to healthcare, and also because of concerns about confidentiality and the ethics of consent, a

[14] www.ncepod.org.uk. Previously published annually as two separate Enquiries – into Maternal Deaths, and into Stillbirths and Deaths in Infancy. The 2005 report can be downloaded in full from www.cemach.org.udk/publications/CEMACHPerinatalMortality ReportApril2005.pdf

[15] www.ncepod.org.uk. Previously published annually as the National Confidential Enquiry into Perioperative Deaths. The 2005 report can be downloaded in full from www.ncepod.org.uk/2005.htm

group of senior decision-makers at NICE announced provisional plans to rid the Confidential Enquiries of patients' stories.

Clinicians weren't sure that this was a good idea, and I was invited to join a group of them in trying to persuade NICE to change its mind. Stories, we argued, were invariably the most interesting parts of an otherwise dismally dull document. Reading a story about a real 29-year-old woman who had died of a real postpartum haemorrhage provided a far more salutary lesson for clinical staff and managers than an algorithm that stated what action to take when a hypothetical patient's blood pressure drops below X. But the argument was made that stories about individuals are always anecdotal, and hence might 'bias' the reader through the distortions inherent in the story form.[16] Far better to let the experts distil out the key points for individuals (for example, what skills professionals should have) and organisations (for example, what equipment should be available) and list them as a clear set of bullet points. Finally, suggested an adviser at NICE, stories are only really useful if they are employed to make a very simple point, otherwise the reader may get lost in idiosyncratic and irrelevant detail.

Several of us disagreed with this. Stories, as I have argued elsewhere in this book, are useful for precisely the opposite reasons – they embrace complexity, they elude simple, rational explanations, and their contribution to the debate can rarely be reduced to bullet points. A consultant obstetrician told the story of a teenage girl who had frozen to death in the grounds of a hospital after being discharged late in the afternoon following a miscarriage. Apparently no one – or at least no one on duty at the time – had known that this unfortunate young woman did not have a home to go back to. What is the 'clear learning point' of this case? What is the 'simple message for the organisation'? What instruction, algorithm or risk management protocol might meaningfully replace this story?

The answer is that the story will have different meanings – and different learning points – for different individuals (those with different clinical and management roles in the NHS, social workers, police) and different organisations (hospitals, primary care organisations, advocacy groups). If we were to release this story (for example, by publishing it in the *British Medical Journal*, or even in *The Sun*), I predict that it would be shared, and its meaning negotiated, in a thousand different ways in organisations up and down the country, from the boardroom to the locker room, by people

[16] *See* previous chapter, page 41, for a counter-argument to the risk of sharing 'wrong' stories.

who have been moved by the tragedy and want to do something to prevent a comparable one from occurring locally. The more the story is told in different contexts and settings, the greater will be the diversity of triggers to collective action. And the more likely one group is to come up with a transferable good idea for meeting the needs of disempowered and vulnerable patients.

In April 2005, responsibility for the Confidential Enquiries was taken over by the National Patient Safety Agency (NPSA), who produced a policy on the use of vignettes in October 2005. This policy acknowledged the previously mixed opinion on the use of vignettes, and emphasised that the NPSA upheld the general principle of using stories for illustrative purposes. The authors cautioned against the indiscriminate inclusion of vignettes, which might prove 'dangerous'. According to the policy, vignettes should mainly be used to illustrate commonly occurring scenarios for which there is good evidence for a particular 'best practice'. 'Lengthy, drifting, unstructured or repetitive text' was also discouraged. This policy, although far more accommodating than we had feared after the 2004 meeting at NICE, is still somewhat ambivalent about the usefulness of stories – especially when balanced against their 'dangers'. Whatever the next instalment in this particular policy story may be, I hope that someone, somewhere, will have the foresight to allocate funds for systematic research into the use of vignettes in policy documents. Which brings me to the chapter on narrative research.

Chapter Five

Stories and research

```
047 D  I'm going to give you something called Augmentin
048     it's a little white bullet  ( . )
049     if you take them three times a day ( . )
                                          [
050 P                                     mhm
051 D  and we'll see if it helps you
052 P  okay that's lovely [coughs briefly]
053 D  anything else?
054     ( . )
055 P  uh ( . ) dya dya oh is it Dyazide? ( . )
056     the ( . ) water tablets I'm on?
057 D  you take those regularly?
058 P  yeah every day ( . )
059     now I always take them in the morning but ( . )
060     would it be all right to take them in the night? ( . )
061     you know because oh [sighing]
062     it drives me mad you know
063     cos I ( . ) pass water so much=
064 D  =course you do=
065 P  =and as I say if I'm on holiday I think well
066     I don't want to be running into the toilet all the time
067 D  why are you taking ( . ) water tablets?
068 P  because I'm on HRT?
069 D  o yeah=
070 P  =um ( . ) clif clif cilafin is it? well I've got enough of those ( . )
                      [
071 D                 mmm: mm
072 P  but I wanted the er Seroxat
073     the antidepressant tablets please
074 D  you take those do you?
075 P  yeah
```

Transcript of doctor–patient consultation, with conversation
analysis annotation.[17]
Reproduced with authors' permission (Elwyn & Gwyn, 1999).

[17] *See* Box 5.2, page 75, for a key to the notation.

If, as I argued in Chapter One, storytelling is the perspectival and rhetorical presentation of events and actions through the use of metaphor, embellishment and other literary devices, and if research is the systematic generation of knowledge through the application of rigorous, repeatable and standardised methods, many scientists would say that there is precious little overlap between them. They would be wrong. Like all qualitative research, narrative techniques provide the opportunity to generate insights that cannot be gained using the traditional tools of the quantitative researcher (measurement and experimentation). The task of justifying qualitative research in general is beyond the scope of this book, but if you are unsure about this territory I strongly recommend that you read a general introductory text before you consider narrative in particular (Atkinson *et al.*, 2003).

In this chapter I shall discuss six distinct methodological approaches to the use of narrative in research – narrative interview, naturalistic story-gathering, discourse analysis, case study, action research and meta-narrative systematic review. For each I shall discuss the rationale behind the approach, outline the method (including how data might be analysed) and briefly highlight its strengths and limitations.[18] The six approaches are summarised and contrasted in Table 5.1 on pages 68–9. Despite their differences, all of these approaches have in common some key defining features of research, whose application to narrative-based studies is summarised in Box 5.1.

Box 5.1: When should a study using narrative be classified as research?

The following questions should inform this complex judgement.

1 Did the investigator(s) collect, interpret, collate or present the story/stories with the intention of answering a clear and focused research question?
2 Did the investigator(s) use a recognisable methodological approach (such as narrative interview, ethnography, multi-method case study or action research)?
3 Was the approach applied rigorously and transparently? Consider

---

[18] I have previously presented four of these approaches in a paper co-authored with Jill Russell and Deborah Swinglehurst (Greenhalgh *et al.*, 2005c). I am grateful to the publisher and my co-authors for permission to reproduce and adapt sections of it here.

aspects such as sampling frame, choice of instruments or tools, method of data collection, method of analysis, and so on.

4 Did the investigator(s) demonstrate reflexive awareness in all aspects of the research process and the researcher role?

5 Was there an identifiable unit of analysis (e.g. the person, the incident, the dialogue, the team, the organisation, the patient journey)?

6 Was there a competent and transparent attempt to analyse empirically collected data using a recognised theoretical framework? In other words, did the researchers go beyond 'letting the stories speak for themselves'?

Narrative interview

Personal stories are readily collected and, for reasons explained in Chapter One, effectively convey the experience of illness, suffering, caring and dying. As I indicated in Chapter Four, they can also provide a vivid window on to the healthcare system within which people's illness experiences are embedded. Examples of research based on narrative interview include Scott Murray's study of end-of-life care based on the narratives of people dying from lung cancer or heart failure (Murray *et al.*, 2002), and my own team's study of the experience of diabetes in Bangladeshi patients (Greenhalgh *et al.*, 1998). As well as published research papers, it is worth noting the DIPEX (Database of Individual Patient Experience) project – an ambitious initiative to collect and systematically collate and index a wide range of narrative interviews from patients of different ages, ethnic backgrounds and illness experiences (see www.dipex.org.uk). So far DIPEX covers a number of different cancers, hypertension, sexual health problems and depression, and it also has a separate website of illness narratives from teenagers. Because the narratives have been collected in a research context with full informed consent, they provide an important archive of material with the potential to be analysed by other research teams at a later date.[19]

[19] Another similar initiative (whose emphasis, I believe, is less on developing a research database and more on providing digital resources for professional development of healthcare staff) is the Patient Voices project (www.patientvoices.org.uk).

Table 5.1: Approaches to the use of narrative in research

Approach	Operational definition	Unit of analysis and analytic approach	Main research methods	Intended output of research	Example
1 Narrative interview	Researcher collects and studies illness stories from patients or stories of professional practice from healthcare staff	Individual narrative, analysed for structure, coherence and meaning in a particular social context	Unstructured or semi-structured interview	Understanding of the illness and healthcare experiences of patients and the identity and practice of healthcare staff	(Murray *et al.*, 2002)
2 Naturalistic story-gathering	Researcher becomes a fieldworker immersed in an organisation or group so as to collect 'real' stories in informal space and interpret them in context	Organisational subgroup (e.g. junior nurses). Analysed for subtleties in individuals' and groups' different interpretations of the same event/action over time	Ethnography	Thick description of organisational culture and how it influences particular behaviours and choices of individuals	(Timmons, 2001)
3 Discourse analysis	Researcher studies a range of data (for example, transcripts of conversations) to identify the prevailing ideologies and power relationships which shape and constrain the use of language by individuals	The text, embedded in a set of interpersonal power relationships and a macro-level social context (e.g. organisation, professional group, society)	Micro-analysis of text in context (e.g. a conversation transcript analysed for choice of words, use of silence, pauses, intonation, turn taking and non-verbal interjections such as coughing or standing up)	Insights into how knowledge, truth, morality and normal behaviour are defined and enacted in a particular organisational or social context	(Mishler, 1984; Iedema *et al.*, 2006)

4 Organisational case study	Researcher presents an account of an organisational change initiative in the form of a detailed story	'The case' (the organisation or part of it), analysed for complex and dynamic influences on key events and processes	Multiple qualitative and quantitative methods (e.g. interviews, questionnaires, documentary analysis)	Detailed description of 'the case' as a context for events, plus chronological account of particular events as they unfolded during the study	(Thor et al., 2004)
5 Action research	Researcher works with participants to develop a shared perspective on the problem and its causes, and to plan and implement action	Group of participants, analysed for development and enactment of shared meanings/purpose	Continuous cycle of participation and reflection by team of researcher(s) and participants	Action intended to change (social drama)	(Bate, 2004)
6 Meta-narrative approach to systematic review	Researcher studies published papers to identify the overarching 'storylines' of how different research traditions unfolded	Research tradition, analysed for concepts, theories, methods and instruments as well as how and why it unfolded over time	'Snowball' search strategies, chronological ordering and interpretation of scientific publications	Sense making of scientific endeavour; rich picture of complex topic areas as differently framed and investigated by different research traditions	(Greenhalgh et al., 2005b)

In narrative interview, the researcher invites the participant to 'tell what happened', and allows them to speak uninterrupted until the story ends. The interview may be semi-structured (driven by a series of questions set out in advance) or unstructured (conducted in a more emergent, conversational style). In either case, prompts should only be used to preserve the flow of the story (for example, 'how did you feel at that point?' or 'what happened next?'). The researcher might invite ideas for change in the form of a different ending to the story (for example, 'if you went through that experience again, what would make it easier for you?').

Narrative interviews are qualitative data, and on one level they can be approached using any mainstream method for analysing text. But narrative analysis per se takes the story as a whole, rather than segments of text, as its focus. Muller describes five overlapping stages of narrative analysis – entering the text (reading and preliminary coding to gain familiarity), interpreting (finding connections in the data through successive readings and reflection), verifying (searching the text and other sources for alternative explanations and confirmatory and disconfirming data), representing (writing up an account of what has been learned) and illustrating (selecting representative quotes) (Muller, 1999).

These analytical stages can be approached through one of several disciplinary lenses. All of them share what Muller calls 'the focus on the broad contours of the story' – that is, the context in which it is told, its structure, the dynamics of how plot unfolds, and any patterns that emerge from multiple stories about the same event. Riessman, for example, suggests that narratives can be analysed conversationally (as teller–listener dialogue), performatively (as drama) or politically (the unfolding of events is seen as constrained by prevailing social and institutional norms; *see* section on discourse analysis below) (Riessman, 2001). As I explained in Chapter One, Frank uses a literary framework to classify illness narratives into four basic categories, namely 'restitution', 'tragedy', 'quest' and 'chaos' (Frank, 1998).

The main strength of the narrative interview is its inherent subjectivity. A frequent theme in classical literature (consider *Great Expectations* or *The Grapes of Wrath*) is the struggle of society's underdogs against social injustice or institutional incompetence. Perhaps for this reason, the narrative interview comes into its own when considering the perspective of disadvantaged groups such as the socially excluded, the seriously ill and the very old. But the perspectival nature of stories is potentially a major limitation when they are used as research data. Furthermore, as I emphasised in Chapter Two, a story is an interaction – an artistic and rhetorical performance for an audience who (actively or passively) shape the telling. The narrative interview has been described as *'practical production, the meaning of which is accomplished at the intersection of the interaction of interviewer and respondent'* (Fontana & Frey, 2005). A different interviewer, on a different day, will never be able to collect the 'same' story from a respondent.

The challenge of narrative research is not to 'control for' the inherent subjectivity, inconsistency and emotionality of stories, but to capture these phenomena as data and interpret them appropriately. Gabriel offers some sound methodological advice:

> *'Joining the postmodern choirs of ever smaller voices does little credit to academic research. Disentangling these voices, understanding them, comparing them, . . . questioning them, testing them and qualifying them – these seem to me to be essential judging qualities that mark research into storytelling and narratives as something different from the acts of storytelling and narration themselves . . . It is the researcher's task not merely to celebrate the story or the narrative but to seek to use it as a vehicle for accessing deeper truths than the truths, half-truths and fictions of undigested personal experience.'*
>
> (Gabriel, 2004)

The process of 'accessing deeper truths' is not straightforward, and narrative research should not be equated with privileging the judgement of the researcher over that of the informant. The validity of the research process rests heavily on evidence of the researcher's reflexive awareness. Aristotle's definition of good literature is that it has a powerful emotional impact on the reader (Aristotle, 1996b). The researcher must acknowledge and engage with this emotional dimension – thus turning sympathy, joy, revulsion and even 'mixed emotions' into research data. As in all qualitative research, there should also be a transparent account of how the researcher decided what aspects of the story to include and exclude as data, and how inferences were made. For a more in-depth discussion of methodological rigour in narrative interviewing, see these methodological texts: Gubrium & Holstein, 1998; Gabriel, 2000; Riessman, 2001; Fontana & Frey, 2005.

Naturalistic story-gathering

As I suggested in the previous chapter, stories told informally in organisations may be especially valuable for accessing that elusive composite of shared values and meaning systems that comprises organisational culture. The anthropologist Clifford Geertz puts it thus:

> 'Believing, with Max Weber, that man is an animal suspended in webs of significance he himself has spun, I take culture to be those webs, and the analysis of it to be therefore not an experimental science in search of law but an interpretive one in search of meaning.'
>
> (Geertz, 1973)

This semiotic (meaning-based) view of organisational culture is strongly echoed by leading organisational researchers. Gabriel highlights the fact that stories exchanged by people in organisations have multiple functions in the creation of meaning – they variously inform, entertain, warn, advise, justify, explain, reassure, console, educate, sustain and transmit ideas or values, and draw moral lessons (Gabriel, 2000). Boje has observed that informal stories in organisations are generally multi-authored (with different members alternating the role of teller and listener), highly reflexive (i.e. the past is continually re-created and re-interpreted in the light of the present), dialogical (i.e. the narrative is co-constructed through a dynamic interaction between each teller and listener), and often allusory and fragmented (emerging 'in bits' rather than as fully formed narratives with a fixed cast of characters) (Boje, 1991).

Given these subtleties, the complexities of organisational culture will be inaccessible to the researcher who arrives with a tape recorder and only collects data in formal narrative interviews. Naturalistic enquiry, in which researchers undergo 'immersion in the field' to study actors in their own environment, relatively free from intervention or control, offers scope to produce what Geertz has called 'thick description' – that is, multi-layered interpretation of social actions in context (Geertz, 1973). The main data source for such enquiry consists of the stories and story fragments exchanged in informal interaction with organisational members (and, in the case of service organisations, with its users). The researcher must of course be selective in deciding which of the hundreds of stories heard during the course of the fieldwork to capture as data, and also in assigning the status of 'story' to what might be no more than a sentence – and (as with ethnography in general) the naive or incompetent researcher will lack the skill and sensitivity to select appropriately.

In one variant of the naturalistic approach, the researcher is appointed from within the organisation rather than from an external research team – an example of auto-ethnography (Jones, 2005). In another variant, known as applied ethnography, the researcher explicitly feeds their ethnographic findings back into the organisation in order to effect change (Chambers, 2005).

The principles of narrative analysis set out on page 70 are also pertinent to the analysis of stories gathered in naturalistic settings. Close analysis of the stories as texts will not, of course, be possible if they have been recorded second-order as retrospective field notes (as is usual practice in ethnography). However, collecting and interpreting particular stories within a wider ethnographic study of the organisation gives the researcher a rich context within which to interpret their significance. Paul Atkinson has strongly criticised the conventional narrative interview as charac-terised by *'an extraordinary absence of social context, social action, and social interaction [and] . . . remarkably little sense of how narratives are forged in face-to-face interaction or how they are elicited in given social contexts'* (Atkinson, 1997). In other words, Atkinson sees a very positive trade-off between the accuracy with which the text of a narrative is recorded and the richness (and hence validity) of the context in which it is captured.

A naturalistic approach enables the collection and comparison of multiple stories about a single issue or event. As the 'toilet-paper' story on page 52 illustrated, organisational 'fictions' have much to contribute to the thick description of culture advocated by Geertz. The limitations of naturalistic story-gathering are both practical and theoretical. 'Prolonged immersion in the field' holds little currency with today's cost-conscious research funders – and in any case, change initiatives may move too quickly. Being an 'insider' to a story of organisational change has both advantages (in-depth knowledge and understanding of issues, rich social networks, mutual trust, timeliness, a longitudinal perspective, ability to effect change and integrate research with development) and disadvantages (lack of critical distance, a specific role in the organisation, prejudices arising from past personal experience, lack of knowledge of the wider context). These issues are discussed further by Winter and colleagues (Winter & Munn Giddings, 2001). For a more detailed methodology of ethnography in general, see Geertz (1973), and for further information on organisational ethnography, see Gabriel (2000) or Boje (2001).

Discourse analysis

There are many theoretical variants of and methodological approaches to discourse analysis in the academic literature, most of which are beyond the scope of this book.[20] In the sense in which I want to present it here, discourse analysis is the study of the overarching meta-narratives and symbol systems in which a particular story is embedded. It is concerned with understanding language within its wider social, historical, political and cultural context. In particular, it considers how prevailing ideologies and power relationships shape and constrain the use of language by individuals (including what comes to be defined as knowledge, morality, truth and normal behaviour). Michel Foucault, for example, believed that *'nothing has any meaning outside of discourse'* – in other words, that the meaning of everything we say and do depends not only on the words available to us in language but also on the symbolic meaning in a particular culture of (for example) a doctor's white coat, a bridal gown, or a Thanksgiving dinner (Foucault, 1973).

We tell particular stories in particular situations because those are the only stories we have the power to tell. Thus the stories we tell (and, even more so, the silences and absent characters in our stories) say much about the nature of our oppression. Key writers on discourse analysis include Foucault, Jaques Derrida (Derrida, 1974) and Jurgen Habermas (Habermas, 1987). All have a radical reputation as critical theorists – that is, as academics who seek fundamentally to challenge prevailing assumptions and ideologies about the nature of society and our freedom within it. For an overview of critical theory as applied to health, see Graham Scambler's excellent book (Scambler, 2001).

Almost all approaches to discourse analysis share an emphasis on the 'deconstruction' of the text – that is, a standing back and considering, usually from a political–ideological perspective, of what is the wider symbolic meaning of the story being told, perhaps through questions such as 'Why did the author use this word or phrase at this point?' or 'Why did the author fail to mention X?'.

---

[20] A colleague who read through the first draft of this book, and who knows far more about discourse analysis than I do, was concerned that I am here presenting only one of many 'takes' on this heterogeneous field, and that experts would disagree with some of the simplifications in this chapter. If you are interested in this fascinating field (as PhD students often are), the chapter 'Definitions of discourse – a sketchy overview' in Maggie MacLure's *Discourses in Educational and Social Research* is a particularly accessible overview of this complex literature (MacLure, 2003).

A classic research study in discourse analysis is Eliot Mishler's analysis of doctor–patient consultations, in which (using conversation analysis, but framed within a theoretical framework from Habermas) he contrasted the 'voice of the lifeworld' (the familiar, knowable space of family and social interaction) with the 'voice of medicine' (the imposed and largely unfamiliar realm of medical institutions, rules and structures that provide the framework in which the consultation takes place) (Mishler, 1984). Mishler demonstrated that doctors (acting unwittingly as agents of the system) unconsciously exclude the lifeworld by repeatedly failing to acknowledge or respond to patients' descriptions of personal and social issues, and by exerting power over the use of time and space in the consultation. Mishler has taken pains to distance himself from the extreme position taken by some discourse analysts – what he calls *'the poststructuralist view of a disembodied* Discourse *or grand master narrative that ''speaks'' through the person'* (Mishler, 1999). Although individual narratives (and dialogues) are situated within these wider discourses, they are not, Mishler claims, mechanistically determined by them.

Box 5.2: Symbols used in conversation analysis, reproduced with permission of the authors (Elwyn & Gwyn, 1999)

- Brackets containing a stop (.) indicate a pause of less than two seconds.
- Numerals in round brackets indicate the length in seconds of other pauses.
- Square brackets [ ] contain relevant contextual information or unclear phrases.
- Italicised square brackets *[.]* describe a non-verbal utterance.
- The symbol [in between lines of dialogue indicates overlapping speech.
- <u>Underlining</u> signifies emphasis.
- An equals sign = means that the phrase is contiguous with the preceding phrase without pause.
- A colon : indicates elongation of the preceding sound.
- D is the doctor.
- P is the patient.

The specific technique used by Mishler to study how narratives are situated within wider social discourses was conversation analysis – that is, the in-depth examination of naturally occurring talk. As illustrated by the excerpt on page 65 (Elwyn & Gwyn, 1999), in conversation analysis the dialogue is reproduced down to the last 'um', and annotated using a standard set of symbols (*see* Box 5.2). Intonations (for example, a rise or fall in tone at the end of a sentence), interruptions, pauses, overlapping speech and non-verbal interjections (such as coughing) are all highlighted, thereby revealing the micro-dynamics of the interaction.

The analysis of the annotated transcript is a painstaking task of interpreting each syllable in context, as in this extract:

> *'The cough (052) functions as a discourse marker, signalling the speaker's wish not to terminate the interaction. The doctor's next utterance "anything else?" is characteristic of doctors' pre-closing moves in medical interactions, but leaves such closure to the patient. The patient (P) is in a position to allow closure or to shift to a new topic. She opts to respond (055), after a false start, first with a pause, then a request for "water tablets". The pause here indicates that there is to be a new topic, but it precludes any accusation of indecent haste. The patient does not wish to be perceived simply as itemising a shopping list. The ritual of correct timing is necessary to maintain the necessary gravity accorded to the ceremony of consultation and prescription. Although the pause lasts less than two seconds, its significance should not be underestimated.'*
>
> (Elwyn & Gwyn, 1999)

The emergence of the research tradition applying discourse analysis to doctor–patient interactions marked an important shift in the study of the biomedical consultation – from a consideration of its structural elements (identifying, for example, 'establishing a relationship', 'determining the reason for attendance', 'performing an examination', 'considering the findings', 'deciding on treatment' and 'termination') (Byrne & Long, 1976) to determining how meaning is not only co-constructed through dialogue but also shaped by external influences. As the excerpt on page 65 (and also the fictitious example of a doctor–patient dialogue described in Chapter Two, page 19) illustrates, conversation generates story because the presence of an audience aids (and stimulates) narration (Bakhtin, 1984). But the words exchanged between doctor and patient (*'if I'm on holiday I think well I don't want to be running into the toilet all the time'*, *'why are you taking water tablets?'*, *'because I'm on HRT'*) are themselves shaped by power relationships (who is seen to be 'in charge' of the consultation) and social expectations (the extent to which a middle-aged woman would be expected to argue with the doctor). The patient raises a lifeworld issue – the inconvenience of running to the toilet all the time when taking diuretics – but the doctor, by ignoring this story fragment, deems this aspect of the problem 'off limits'. He steers the conversation back to the biomedical agenda (the reason why the tablets were prescribed), and the patient meekly follows his lead by responding in the 'discourse of medicine'.

Discourse analysis does not only apply to conversations. For example, Iedema and colleagues used discourse analysis to analyse critical incident reports in the study described in the previous chapter (*see* page 56) (Iedema *et al.*, 2006), and one of my colleagues is currently using discourse analysis to deconstruct the unfolding 'story' in a succession of government policy documents. The common feature of all these approaches is an attempt to critically deconstruct whatever text(s) have been chosen as the unit of analysis.

Deconstruction is an interpretive and thus highly contestable act, as anyone who has had a discussion about the political undertones of a play will vouch. There are many doctors (especially, one is tempted to suggest, old-fashioned and unreflexive ones) who would contest Mishler's assertion that medical consultations are an unequal power contest between the voice of medicine and the voice of the lifeworld. Similarly, Iedema's assertion that critical incident reporting by doctors is powerfully influenced by organisational meta-discourse is one of many competing interpretations that could be placed on his dataset. At the end of the day, we must judge these researchers' conclusions as we judge any story – by their coherence, authenticity, persuasiveness and explanatory value (*see* page 9).

One of the main strengths of discourse analysis is its potential to link micro-level processes (for example, the verbal exchange in a patient–GP consultation, or the scribbling of a report form following a medical disaster or near miss) with macro-level ones (for example, the social, political and economic system within which patients consult and medical mishaps occur). Its main limitation (in the eyes of its critics) is its inherent tendency to politicise scientific data and suggest only macro-level solutions (such as fundamental changes in the nature of social institutions). Whether or not you feel drawn to try discourse analysis yourself will probably be partly determined by your ideological position in relation to the critical theory agenda.

Case study[21]

Case study research considers a social system ('case') in context and explores it in sufficient detail to illuminate relationships and processes and provide insights into *why* particular events unfold as they do. Like ethnography (with which it overlaps considerably), case study involves detailed, reflexive fieldwork leading to rich, authentic description. It requires the prospective in-depth investigation of an organisation, team or other complex social grouping using multiple methods – typically a combination of formal interviews, focus groups, participant observation, and collection of contemporaneous materials (minutes of meetings, emails, memos, etc.).

Constructing a case study requires considerable judgement and skill. The elements of the case must be iteratively defined through a sequence of sampling (to identify somewhere to start), progressive focusing (to refine and systematically explore what has been sampled), theorising (about interactions within the arbitrarily defined case and across the boundary with the world beyond it), analysing (testing how well the data fit the theory) and interpreting (deriving meaning from the data) (Yin, 1994; Stake, 1996). As I argued in the previous chapter, organisations are complex, containing much social action (and a considerable amount of trouble), so in practice most organisational case studies get analysed and written up in a story-like way. A case study is generally based on a large, heterogeneous, dynamic and complex collection of empirical data, each component of which will first need to be analysed separately (for example, quantitative data statistically, qualitative data thematically) before being woven into a higher-order interpretation of the whole picture and how and why it has changed through time.

'Storying' the case – that is, constructing a chronological, emplotted account of the key actions and events – is a way of selecting which data to focus on and which to omit. It is also a way of drawing meaning from different data sources and making causal links between aspects of the case – either tentatively, as hypotheses to be tested in further research, or more

---

[21] We must distinguish true case study research, which can take years to produce, from the much commoner *case report*, in which one or more members of a team tell a personal story about their initiative and its impact.

firmly, as lessons or conclusions (if the links are particularly strong and plausible). In practice, organisational case studies tend to be the product of several researchers working together over months or years, and the task of processing, interpreting and integrating the data into a coherent story is achieved through interaction between team members – especially the repeated exchange and negotiation of stories.

Stake draws on previous researchers (Van Maanen, 1988) to suggest four approaches to storying that researchers may use to present in-depth case studies:

1 realist tales – a direct, matter-of-fact portrait, a chronological or bio-graphical development of the case
2 confessional tales – the researcher's personal account of coming to know the case and the challenges that they faced
3 impressionist tales – a sequential description of several major compo-nents of the case, *'personalised accounts of fleeting moments of fieldwork case in dramatic form'*
4 illustrative tales – the use of vignettes (storied episodes) to illustrate particular aspects of the case.

In all of these approaches, a good case study researcher, like a good storyteller, will use literary devices to place emphasis and convey surprises and ambiguities, and will 'zoom in' judiciously to analyse the behaviour of individuals within (and as influenced by) the wider system. Once again, an important criterion for judging the rigour of a case study is evidence of the researchers' reflexive awareness and the transparency of their infer-ences from the data.

Case study has been described as 'strong in reality' – that is, as having high potential for validity within the confines of the case itself (Stake, 1996). But researchers who have been raised on the conventional hierarchy of evidence (with randomised controlled trials at the top and anecdote at the bottom) often find it hard to identify much value in case study research. The $64,000 question might be put as follows. To what extent does case study trade external validity (i.e. direct transferability to other contexts) for internal coherence and richness, and (conversely) to what extent will a detailed and systematic analysis of one unique 'case' give us robust, transferable lessons for application elsewhere?

This question is much debated among case study theorists (see, for example, a recent compilation by Gomm *et al.*, 2000). Yin takes the conventional scientific view that a case is only meaningful as a member of a sociological family of cases which provide the analytical framework to understand it (*'previously developed theory is used as a template with which to compare the empirical results of case studies'*) (Yin, 1994). Stake, in contrast, argues from an interpretive perspective that the case is meaningful in its own right (what he calls *'the intrinsic study of the valued particular'*) (Stake, 1996). May, quoted in Simons, describes how his understanding of trees was changed forever when he saw a painting by Cézanne (Simons, 1996). The tree in the painting was not statistically representative of trees in general, nor did it contain features present in every tree. Nevertheless, the qualities that Cézanne had illuminated in his particular tree enabled the author to see every subsequent tree through new eyes. Simons argues that the hallmark of a good case study is this metaphorical (rather than scientific) generalisability.

A good worked example of case study is a five-year study by Thor and colleagues of an ambitious quality improvement initiative in an acute hospital, based on 'learning facilitators' who helped a total of 93 project teams (Thor *et al.*, 2004). The researchers attributed the success of the facilitators to allowing each clinical team to remain in charge of their ideas and adopting a supporting role that comprised:

1 providing feedback on ideas and progress
2 helping with demanding (and sometimes menial) tasks
3 developing specialist skill and experience in quality improvement
4 taking responsibility for small practicalities, such as refreshments for meetings.

Arguably, the validity of this case does not rest on (nor would it be enhanced by) the presence of a 'control group' or 'comparative cases' – it rests on the authenticity of the observations and interpretations about what happened in *this* case. Of course, we cannot extrapolate these findings to every quality improvement project (for example, we cannot say that providing cookies at meetings will always improve the quality of decisions). But we can learn a general lesson from a facilitation approach characterised by 'mucking in' and taking account of specific contextual features (in this case, that meetings were often held over mealtimes).

In-depth case study is labour-intensive and usually takes years to produce (not an endearing characteristic in a climate where researchers are judged by the number of papers they write and the speed with which they publish). Another potential limitation is that because of the detailed contextual information necessary to understand the case, organisations (and the individuals within them) may be identifiable. Glyn Elwyn's team has described a way of fictionalising organisational case studies by first abstracting the key themes from a sample of cases (for example, high user expectations, lack of cash, external policy mandates, and so on), and then writing a new story that includes all of these key themes (Elwyn *et al.*, 2002).

Action research

Action research – defined as *'a mutual learning process within which people work together to discover what the issues are, why they exist, and how they might be addressed'* (Bate, 2000) – has an important narrative (performative) dimension. It is usually presented as a cycle or spiral composed of successive phases (identify focus of enquiry → gather baseline data → analyse data to generate hypotheses → plan action → gather data to evaluate impact of action → shift to new focus of enquiry) (Waterman *et al.*, 2001). The link between action research and narrative is rarely made, probably because the performative element of narrative (*see* page 9) is not widely acknowledged.

As I explained in the previous chapter (*see* page 54), knowledge-based theories of organisational change centre on the need for the members to make sense of change efforts by assimilating them into their cognitive schemata, and to embody the change effort as part of their own individual and professional identity. In the previous chapter (*see* page 54), I described an example of action research directed at organisational change, namely Paul Bate's quality improvement initiative in a 'failing' UK NHS hospital trust, in which the mechanism for change was the development and enactment of what might be called a change drama (Bate, 2004). My own team's work in developing the 'sharing stories' intervention described in Chapter Three (*see* page 33) was also an example of action research (Greenhalgh *et al.*, 2005a).

A great strength of action research is that it does what it says on the can – it is inherently action-oriented and seeks to get things done that benefit the participants directly. Collective sense making of past and present events feeds into creative, collaborative action. For this reason, an action research approach can sometimes be ethically justified in situations where other designs may be more difficult to defend (for example, when working to improve services for disempowered groups). The main limitation of action research is that it is a highly specialised and intensive approach of which there are as yet few rigorously conducted examples in the mainstream medical literature. Perhaps for this reason, it is almost impossible to secure funding for action research from biomedical research bodies, although many grant-giving bodies offer 'development' funds that can be channelled into action research.

Meta-narrative systematic review

A systematic review is a review of the literature that has been conducted using an explicit, rigorous and auditable method. For most people in the biomedical field, that means adopting the methods set out in the *Cochrane Reviewers' Handbook 4.2.2* (Cochrane Collaboration, 2004), which describes how to search electronic databases, apply 'critical appraisal checklists' to papers, extract data and perform the statistics for meta-analysis. In Chapter Two (*see* page 24) I argued that the science of evidence-based medicine was built on a myth – that the judgements required in clinical practice are fundamentally technical ones. The science of systematic review, as perpetrated by what might be called the 'hardliners' of the Cochrane Collaboration, is built on a similar myth – that the judgements required to summarise and synthesise research findings from different primary studies can also be reduced to a series of technical decisions and processes.

As I have argued at length elsewhere (Greenhalgh *et al.*, 2005b), this assumption is only reasonable when a simple research question has been addressed in a similar way by several teams (for example, when a reviewer seeks to summarise the findings of half a dozen studies that all tested the effect of drug X on clinical outcome Y in disease Z). When the research we seek to summarise addresses complex fields of enquiry and 'wicked' questions (that is, those with no simple or unambiguous answer, such as often happens in policy-making research), the nature of judgement is fundamentally different – it shifts from being predominantly technical to being predominantly interpretive. Here is a passionate attack from a professor of education who sees her business as interpretive judgement:

'[Conventional systematic review] assumes that evidence can be extracted intact from the texts in which it is embedded, and "synthesised" in a form that is impervious to ambiguities of context, readers' interpretations of writers' arguments (i.e. bias). Most significantly of all, systematic review systematically degrades the central acts of reviewing: namely <u>reading</u> and <u>writing</u>, and the unreliable intellectual acts that these support, such as interpretation, argument, and analysis. By replacing reading and writing

> *with an alternate lexicon of scanning, screening, mapping, data extraction, and synthesis, systematic review tries to transform reading and writing into accountable acts. It tries to force their clandestine operations – the bits that happen inside people's heads – or in the incorporeal gaps between decoding and comprehension, thought and expression – up into plain view, where they can be observed, quality-controlled and stripped of interpretation or rhetoric.'*
>
> (MacLure, 2005)

A few years ago, I worked with a multi-disciplinary team to undertake a systematic review of the literature on diffusion of innovations in health service organisations (Greenhalgh *et al.*, 2004). It became clear early on that different teams of researchers had all conceptualised 'diffusion of innovations' in different ways. The 400 research papers and 100 chapters listed in our final report had been published in around 350 different journals or books, asked approximately 150 different research questions, used 29 different research designs, and had been summarised in at least six previous systematic reviews (all of which had rejected different primary studies as 'methodologically flawed', combined the data in different ways, and reached different conclusions and recommendations). Halfway through our study, we very nearly handed the money back to our funder on the grounds that the task we had set ourselves was proving impossible.

To cut a long story short, after a considerable intellectual struggle we came up with a new approach to systematic review – meta-narrative review – in which the main unit of analysis was what we called the 'research storyline'. We found that the most sensible way of sorting out our piles of research papers was to group them according to 'who cites whom', 'who reads the same journals' and 'who goes to the same conferences'. We came to see it as crucially important that any group of scientists undertaking any piece of research is consciously building on a particular body of previous research, and that research is conventionally written up as a narrative that begins with 'background' (what particular others have previously shown) and ends with 'discussion' (how this new finding fits into a particular wider picture).

We used Thomas Kuhn's notion of a research tradition (a body of work that shares four things: a conceptual basis, a theory or set of theories, an agreed methodological approach and an accepted set of instruments) (Kuhn, 1962). Kuhn had previously recognised that any scientific finding only makes sense when interpreted within a particular research paradigm. For example, Newtonian physics makes sense if you use the concepts, theories, methods and instruments that Newton himself used, but it becomes 'flawed' when Einsteinian concepts, theories, methods and instruments are applied. Kuhn showed that a research tradition emerges dynamically over time and goes through three key phases – pre-paradigmatic (when 'ideas people' are developing its conceptual and theoretical basis), paradigmatic (a phase of 'systematic puzzle solving' using methods and instruments that are now largely agreed) and post-paradigmatic (when refinements in methods and instruments generate data that cannot be explained by the core concepts and theories of the paradigm, which creates the tension needed for breakaway scientists to start a new paradigm).

Before we applied a narrative approach, the research literature on diffusion of innovations appeared as an incoherent mass of studies in which no researchers were singing from the same hymn sheet. But by looking for research storylines, and sorting the individual papers into time order within each storyline, we were able to unpick 13 distinct research traditions,[22] including rural sociology (the study of what influences farmers to change their agricultural practices), communication studies (the study of the spread of information, especially 'news'), development studies (the study of the adoption, adaptation and use of technology, especially in a development context), guideline implementation studies (the study of why clinicians adopt or fail to adopt best research evidence) and knowledge utilisation studies (the study of how knowledge spreads and becomes embedded in organisations). By first unpicking these separate storylines, and then combining them in a unifying narrative, we were able to build up a rich picture of the research territory relevant to diffusion of innovations in healthcare organisations.

Meta-narrative review is not, of course, a panacea. It is hard work, and because you will uncover multiple perspectives that are by definition incommensurable, the risk of confusion in your own mind or conflict in your research team is high. But I believe that the approach has genuine advantages in certain circumstances – in particular where the scope of a project is broad and the literature diverse, where different groups of scientists have asked different questions and used different research designs to address a common problem, where different groups of practitioners and policy makers have drawn on the research literature in

---

[22] We stopped at 13 research traditions because our funds were limited, but we could probably have gone on and added another 10.

different ways, where 'quality' papers have different defining features in different literatures, and where there is no self-evident or universally agreed process for pulling the different bodies of literature together.[23]

I hope that by talking you through how narrative techniques can be applied in six different research designs, I have illustrated first that storytelling and research can be successfully combined without losing rigour, and secondly that quality standards for doing (and evaluating) narrative research can be developed. This chapter is not intended either as a comprehensive taxonomy of narrative research methods (I can think of three or four other approaches which I could have included, and I've probably forgotten several more) or as a definitive guide to the 'critical appraisal' of narrative-based research studies. All narrative research is inherently dialogic and interpretive, and I leave you with the suggestion that the 'appraisal' of narrative research requires, above all else, a process of interpretation through dialogue. If the ideas presented in this chapter provide a springboard from which further discussion can be launched, I will have achieved a more important objective than having the last word on narrative research myself.

[23] Meta-narrative review was developed from, and has considerable overlap with, the realist approach to systematic review originally developed by Ray Pawson (Pawson, 2002), although he does not place any special emphasis on storylines. Pawson and I have subsequently published together on realist review and highlighted the distinction between these two approaches (Pawson *et al.*, 2005).

Chapter Six

Stories and ethics

In one of the sessions of the 'sharing stories' group for bilingual health advocates, one member of the group arrived very late. She was clearly upset and angry. This was her story. She had spent the morning in a busy outpatient clinic, interpreting in doctor–patient consultations. Mid-morning, she was summoned urgently to the antenatal ward where a non-English-speaking patient, 28 weeks pregnant, was standing in the middle of the ward, screaming. The advocate approached the patient, somewhat nervously at first since the message had been conveyed that she had 'gone mad', and quickly ascertained that a few minutes previously the unfortunate woman had suddenly lost the sight in both eyes. She conveyed this information to the nurses, guided the patient back to her bed, and tried to reassure and comfort her until her husband arrived.

Shortly afterwards, there was a phone call from the outpatient clinic. The advocate was needed to interpret, and the doctors were getting impatient as it was nearly lunchtime. She tried to resist, but the nurses insisted that she must return to the clinic immediately, especially since a provisional diagnosis had now been made and the patient had stopped screaming. They even reminded her that as an outpatient services advocate, she was not employed to hang around on the ward. The advocate, who looked physically exhausted, told the group that she had seen a total of 72 patients that morning, rushing from one room to another in the outpatient clinic as different doctors called on her services. But she couldn't get the pregnant woman out of her mind, and felt that she had failed her.

Story shared in a learning set for bilingual health advocates
(*see* Chapter 3)

In this chapter I shall make three points. First, the *content* of stories raises ethical questions, and that stories (both 'fact' and fiction) are therefore a useful tool for teaching ethics and analysing ethical challenges in our lives and work. Second, the *process* of collecting, analysing, distributing and publishing stories in turn raises other ethical questions – about consent, confidentiality, privacy and the thorny issue of who owns the 'data'. My third point, which runs across both of the first two, is that the distinctive features of the narrative form discussed in previous chapters offer a method for addressing both kinds of ethical question.

Most (perhaps all) of the stories in this book raise ethical issues – such as how to live a good life, how to be a good doctor, good nurse, good patient or good relative, how to balance conflicting professional demands and patients' needs, and so on. The story at the beginning of this chapter is a powerful example. The patient's 'trouble' is particularly dramatic and tragic (she is young, pregnant, alone and confused, and the medical problem is serious, unfair and possibly incurable), the advocate's obligations are especially acute (she is the only actor on the scene who can communicate with the patient, whose sudden blindness has cut her off from important visual cues such as smiling and even from bodily orientation), and the 'system' seems, even more than usual, not to care. Small wonder that the advocate was distressed.

I shall return to this story and its emotional significance shortly, but first I want to digress into fiction to help to illustrate a theoretical point about the nature of ethical judgement. If you have children or grandchildren, and perhaps even if you don't, you may have read JK Rowling's Harry Potter books, which feature the adventures of a trio of teenagers in the splendid context of Hogwarts School of Witchcraft and Wizardry. You may also recall claims by fundamentalist Christians that the Harry Potter books encourage children to dabble in the occult, and should therefore be banned (or even ceremonially burned).[24] Christian parents (and Jewish and Muslim ones, too, for that matter) might understandably feel uneasy about exposing their children to a fictional universe in which the heroes regularly meddle with black magic but where God doesn't ever feature.

As theologian Francis Bridger argues convincingly in *A Charmed Life: The Spirituality of Potterworld*, the fundamentalists' claims are entirely unfounded (Bridger, 2002). The three heroes of the Potter books – Harry, Ron and Hermione – find themselves in a succession of adventures in which the essential recurring storyline is the looming of an evil threat which they alone can avert, so long as they break one or more school rules. The threesome (who are around 11 years old at the start of the first book and will be 18 at the end of the last one) move from what Bridger calls an 'infantile morality' that is based on universal and inflexible rules ('don't tell lies', 'obey the teachers') to a more sophisticated morality in which these rigid rules become rules of thumb to be applied judiciously and in context. You mustn't climb out of the dormitory window in the middle of the night – unless you have good reason to suppose that your actions could prevent the evil Lord Voldemort from destroying the world.

[24] See, for example, www.cuttingedge.org/news/hpmain.html

The magic in Potterworld is, as Bridger astutely observes, not 'black' at all but entirely incidental to the battle between good and evil. The characters use it in the same way that James Bond uses his gadgets – to break through locks or fix a broken broomstick. Whilst the magic used by Harry Potter can be mischievous (he occasionally uses it to make a custard pie fall on an adversary), it is not Satanic, and the real ethical judgements lie elsewhere (should they or shouldn't they truant a lesson to find out more about the dastardly Voldemort?). The Potter plots repeatedly illustrate, in an increasingly sophisticated way as the heroes grow in maturity, the development of moral virtues such as courage, tenacity and loyalty, and the application of these virtues to the 'trouble' caused by the less virtuous characters. Potterworld is thus a highly moral universe from which children (and indeed adults) can learn important lessons about ethical behaviour and judgements (Bridger, 2002). The fundamentalists' converse interpretation is a superb illustration of why abstract principles ('magic is wrong') are no help in complex ethical decision making.[25]

Let us return to the story of the advocate and the newly blind patient. Before I discuss it further, I should remind you that the account as I have depicted it has all the limitations of the narrative form set out elsewhere in this book (*see*, for example, page 71). The original story told orally in the group was perspectival, unverified and (quite possibly) highly selective in what was reported. Whilst I have tried faithfully to recall what was said, I may have remembered things wrongly. It is even possible that the advocate made it up to save face when she arrived late and in tears over some completely different incident, although I have no reason to doubt either her own integrity or that of her story. With those caveats in mind, let us analyse some ethical issues.

The advocate's job description required her to be in the outpatient clinic that morning, and she had no official business being on the ward, because the urgent summons had not followed protocol. Despite this, when we meet the action, the advocate *is* on the ward – and we must take that situation as our starting point for ethical analysis. General ethical principles (such as beneficence, non-maleficence, autonomy and justice) are

[25] If you'd like to go beyond Harry Potter for an example of the use of character and plot in literature to illustrate ethical arguments, Martha Nussbaum makes similar philosophical points (and takes them to a considerably higher intellectual plane) based on the work of such literary giants as Marcel Proust, James Joyce and John Steinbeck (Nussbaum, 2001), and there are several more examples in a recent compilation from Rita Charon's team (Charon & Montello, 2002).

useful rules of thumb, but will not tell us whose needs should take priority for the professional services of the advocate – those of the one patient on the ward or those of the many in the clinic. We can, however, answer this question by considering the ethical problem *as story* (Who are the actors? What has happened so far? What will be the consequences of different courses of action? How do we *feel* about those consequences?). In this particular instance, the needs of the one are acute, urgent, profound and laden with emotion, whereas those of the many are ongoing, non-urgent, relatively minor and we feel relatively impassive about them. In short, the many can wait.

Why, then, was the opposite decision made? Perhaps it was because:

1 the doctors in the outpatient clinic did not know the particularities of the case
2 the nurses on the ward were too junior to make a competent judgement about the meaning of the message 'the advocate is needed urgently'
3 the advocate was trapped in a low-status organisational role in which it would have been considered inappropriate for her to have sought a telephone negotiation with a doctor.

The ward nurses (who might well have been students), as well as taking a naive, mechanistic and institution-focused view of what purpose the advocate's presence was serving (to translate, to remove the woman from the middle of the ward, and to stop her screaming), were applying an infantile morality system – 'always obey the orders of senior doctors' – rather than using the situational judgement of the experienced professional. The system, of course, was not 'uncaring' – it was just the system. But there was, both individually and collectively, a failure to break the general system rules when the story demanded this. And the poor advocate found herself embodying this failure and expressing it in her distraught emotional state.

Two eminent philosophers, Alasdair MacIntyre and Martha Nussbaum, have each presented a more detailed theoretical discussion of why medical ethics must move from rigid universal rules to story-based situational judgements that not only have a particular and specific past history and present context, but also have a particular set of future consequences (MacIntyre, 1982; Nussbaum, 2001). Their positions contrast sharply with the much more widespread view that general ethical principles can be applied universally and in a logico-deductive way in order to reach a 'rational' decision about what is right (an approach known as principle-based ethics or just 'principalism') (Beauchamp & Childress, 2001).

Principle-based ethics, for example, is the basis of the publication *Duties of a Doctor*, with which most UK doctors are familiar (General Medical Council, 1995).

Perhaps the most crucial distinction between principle-based ethics and narrative ethics is the role of emotion. Principle-based ethics suggests that emotions 'get in the way' of the task of reaching an ethical decision, which should be made objectively and in a standardised manner across cases. Medical students are sometimes taught that they 'mustn't get involved' in the emotional aspects of the cases they see (and that if they do, their decisions will be less ethical). They may also be taught that ethical principles can be applied in the same essentially technical manner as clinical guidelines (as in evidence-based medicine). But in narrative ethics (sometimes known as existential ethics or virtue ethics – or even, in Aristotle's timeless monograph, Nicomachean ethics) (Aristotle, 1996a), the emotional reaction to the case – to the characters, actions and events in the story – is *part of the process* of reaching an ethical decision. It is because we know that the advocate feels angry, frustrated and sad about being torn away from the ward – and because we share some of those emotions – that we uncover the unresolved ethical issues.

In her excellent book *Upheavals of Thought: The Intelligence of Emotions*, philosopher Martha Nussbaum (drawing on Aristotle's *Poetics*) has argued that 'emotions do moral work' – in other words, our emotional reaction to the stories that unfold in our lives is a crucial stimulus for, and component of, ethical action (Nussbaum, 2001). Nussbaum argues that a theory of emotion (take love, anger, jealousy, gratitude, pity or guilt, for example) comprises three key notions – a cognitive appraisal or evaluation of an external object, the idea of one's own flourishing or one's own important goals, and the idea of the salience of external objects (especially other people) in the pursuit of these goals. Emotions, she claims, give body and inner voice to the process of cognitive evaluation of things that are external in relation to the things that are at stake in one's life (or the life of another with whom we identify). Thus defined, emotions have both a narrative dimension (they relate to an ongoing personal story comprising context, plot so far, present trouble and imagined future possibilities) and an ethical one (we feel a particular emotion *because* a particular happening or possibility has been appraised as having a particular type of moral poignancy and a greater or lesser moral value). A life devoid of emotion is a flat plane without form or feature; emotions, argues Nussbaum, produce 'geological upheavals of thought' that transform the flat plane into a rich landscape with height, depth and perspective.

The link between narrative and virtue, according to MacIntyre, is not only that virtues (courage, tenacity, altruism) are demonstrated in specific situations and actions (i.e. through our role in the stories that make up our lives), but also that virtues are *developed* by applying them in specific situations. To return to Harry Potter, it is through the various moral crusades that Harry and his friends undertake that they acquire depth of character and specific virtues. As the pop song goes, Oz never did give nothing to the Tin Man / That he didn't already have – but it took the various exploits of the Yellow Brick Road for the Tin Man to *acquire* the heart that he so desperately sought.

Anne Hudson Jones, who teaches medical ethics to undergraduates in the USA, has described how the study of fictional stories in literature can help students to move beyond the recourse to abstract principles and achieve a richer analysis of the ethics of particular cases. For example:

> *'In both "The Use of Force" [William Carlos Williams] and "Brute" [Richard Seltzer], a physician physically assaults a patient in order to diagnose or treat. The ethical issue is whether such powerful medical paternalism can be justified by appealing to beneficence – that is, by claiming that what the physician did was for the patient's own good. But by attending to the richly evocative language used by the physician-narrators of these stories, readers have the opportunity to learn about more than patient autonomy and physician paternalism. They can learn how ethical principles and arguments may sometimes be used to rationalize unethical behavior that is driven by sexual attraction, anger, or pride.'*
>
> (Jones, 1998)

Jones also makes the point that if medical students can acquire the basic techniques of literary analysis, they can start to use these skills in clinical history taking and also in the evaluation of ethical issues that arise from it. For example, questions like those listed below (which are, of course, at a different level of abstraction) can augment the usual checklist of questions such as 'How long has she had the pain?' and 'What medication is she taking?':

- Who is the narrator?
- Is the narrator reliable?

- From what angle of vision does the narrator tell the story?
- What has been left out of the narrative?
- Whose voice is not being heard and why?
- What kind of language and images does the narrator use?
- What effect does this kind of language have in creating patterns of meaning that emerge from the text?

These 'literary' questions (questions *about* the medical history rather than ones that form part of it) can also be used to interrogate the professional's version of events and compare it with the patient's version. As Anne Hudson Jones and others have pointed out, ethical problems in clinical care are always 'framed' by the actors involved in ways that suggest a particular 'plot'. For example, a cancer patient's decision to take homeopathic treatment rather than undergo chemotherapy might be framed by doctors as non-compliance, denial or confusion, and the patient's character might be presented as flighty, ignorant or stubborn, although this would not, presumably, be the patient's (or the homeopath's) construction of the story. A crucial contribution of the narrative perspective in medical ethics is in mapping the territory and constructing the description of what is conventionally referred to as 'the case'. As Susan Rubin argues in a paper entitled 'Beyond the authoritative voice', the use of the patient's own narrative as the starting point for ethical analysis precludes the clinician (or ethicist) from using his or her own perspective and values to decide what are and are not important components of the 'case' (Rubin, 2002).

In the past ten years it has become commonplace for medical schools to include, either as part of the standard curriculum or as optional modules, the literary study of both illness as depicted in fiction and personal accounts of healthcare experiences. I have no idea whether students who sign up for these courses (and whose assessment includes a humanities-style essay paper in which they are asked to analyse illness narratives as texts) make better ethical judgements or not after they have qualified. I suspect that there would be prohibitive practical constraints on researching this question. Perhaps we will have to take on trust the value of such training and its relative benefits compared with a more conventional use of curriculum time. If you teach students yourself, or if you are a student who would like to change the syllabus of your own medical school to include a narrative perspective on ethics, a good place to start is the Medical Humanities website of the New York University School of Medicine (http://endeavor.med.nyu.edu/lit-med/), which includes a searchable database of suitable literary texts on subjects ranging from prison healthcare to African-Caribbean accounts of sickle-cell crises, and also offers examples of medical humanities curricula from different medical schools throughout the world.

The role of literature in developing the sensibilities and skills needed for the practice of medicine or nursing is not confined to works about illness. Although stories involving doctors (good, bad and indifferent) are clearly of direct value in considering one's own role as a doctor, and patients' stories allow the clinician reader to 'live through' the patient experience, human virtues (and vices) can be illustrated, and human suffering depicted, in stories that include neither doctors nor patients. John Salinsky's book *Medicine and Literature: the Doctor's Companion to the Classics* includes literary critiques of such greats as *Tristram Shandy* (by Sterne), *Madame Bovary* (by Flaubert) and *Anna Karenina* (by Tolstoy) (Salinsky, 2002). Each chapter covers a different literary classic and draws lessons relevant to clinical practice (many of them about clinical ethics). One for your Christmas list!

The final topic I want to cover in this chapter is the ethics of narrative research. The arguments on page 91 on the advantages of narrative ethics over principle-based ethics in clinical decisions can equally well be applied to ethical decisions in research. The arguments are well set out in two articles in a recent compilation on narrative ethics in the special issue of *Health* published in October 2005 (Mattingly, 2005; Riessman, 2005). The issue sprang from an interdisciplinary conference on 'Narrative-Based Medicine'[26] which some colleagues and I organised in Cambridge in 2001. The audience included a high proportion of doctors who were sympathetic to the idea of narrative research but not familiar with its subtleties, and who were more used to attending conventional medical conferences. They were surprised to hear speakers reading unedited accounts of illness narratives in which the individual's identity had not been fully 'anonymised', and to see posters of visual narratives (i.e. photographs) in which the faces of the research participants had not been blacked out (as is standard procedure for pictures in biomedical publications). During the conference, and especially in the informal spaces

[26] If you think I invented this term as a cheap marketing ploy to sell the idea of narrative to a medical audience that was at the time largely preoccupied with evidence-based medicine, you'd be right. Having coined the term 'narrative-based medicine' to get the narrative agenda on the table, I'd now like to see it dropped.

outside the official sessions, heated discussions were held on topics such as consent, confidentiality, privacy, and so on – and these provided the seeds of the special journal issue.

One important theme arising from that conference discussion, which I have already covered in depth above in relation to clinical ethics, is the contextual and specific nature of ethical decisions. No one is suggesting that the *principle* of confidentiality is incorrect, but there are times when it is ethically preferable to breach (or at least to modify the meaning of) that principle. In her Cambridge presentation, Cheryl Mattingly showed a video of the young black child of a poor single mother. The child was dying of a brain tumour following a lengthy period of treatment that had proved unsuccessful. Cheryl gave a highly personal account of getting to know the child and her mother, and of the pair's struggles not just against the unrelenting progress of the tumour, but also against poverty, stigma and the cold objectivity with which some doctors approached the thera-peutic relationship. She described how following the little girl's death (we were shown a clip of the family's home video of the funeral, in which balloons were released and floated up to the sky, to much cheering), her mother had found a new identity in supporting other parents of seriously ill children and had founded a charity in her daughter's name.

As I chaired that session, I remember looking out at a packed conference hall and seeing an entire audience close to tears. The speaker's academic message – about the value of the performative narrative in generating hope in a seemingly hopeless situation – was clear, but the presentation also (I believe) changed our clinical practice. Every health professional in the audience returned to clinical practice humbled by the story of this courageous mother, and more aware of the little things that can make a big difference for patients with terminal illness.

The personal nature of the presentation was not a mistake. Cheryl had not *forgotten* to anonymise or objectify her 'data', nor was she simply being slack about the style of her presentation. Rather, in the course of her research relationship with the child's mother (which was unusually deep and trusting, born of the shared intimacy of repeated ethnographic visits), she became aware that *this* mother did not seek anonymity but its exact opposite – an international platform from which to change the behaviour of doctors towards people like her, so that others in similar situations might be spared a little of the heartache she and her daughter had been through. She had even explicitly asked Cheryl to use her daughter's real name, not a pseudonym, when presenting their case.

Measured by the standards of principle-based ethics (and indeed by many of the biomedical guidelines for presenting 'cases' at research conferences), this example gives grounds for concern. But if the yardstick is narrative ethics, the conclusion is very different. Using MacIntyre's starting point of *'which story or stories do I find myself a part of?'* (MacIntyre, 1982), the researcher decided to assist with the task that the research 'subject' had declared her personal quest. Not only was the 'breach of confidentiality' justified in this particular case for this particular audience, but also an anonymised (and less emotionally evocative) version of the same presentation would surely have been *less* ethical, given whose story (and whose 'data') it was and what was at stake for the surviving character.

Set in the context of a book on narrative, the above arguments probably strike you as more or less convincing. But if you were a member of a biomedical research ethics panel, bound by its conventions, you would probably feel differently. In another article in the special issue of *Health*, Elvi Whittaker describes struggles with what in the USA are called Institutional Research Boards and what we in the UK call Research Ethics Committees (Whittaker, 2005). The dominance of procedure over what most of us would call judgement, the ever-lengthening paper trail required of both researchers and the committees themselves, and the requirement for research participants to be force-fed with small print as part of the process of 'consenting', are all symptoms of a growing bureau-cratisation of research ethics whose origins can, I believe, be traced directly to an over-reliance on principle-based rather than narrative ethics.

Those of us who spend increasing amounts of time in the pursuit of 'ethical approvals' should bear in mind that the people who sit on Research Ethics Committees, and those who make the rules by which they work, are not as individuals devoid of common sense or especially fond of bureaucracy. Nor are they bent on destroying research traditions in clinical fields where contemporary procedures for obtaining consent are impossible (for example, research on people who are suddenly and unexpectedly unconscious) (Warlow, 2005). They are simply taking principle-based ethics to its logical conclusion. Both the mushroom cloud of paperwork and the death of research as we knew and loved it are unanticipated side-effects of their well-meaning intentions.

How can we circumvent this? Nobody is going to read this book (or indeed other publications that have argued similar points; MacIntyre, 1982; Charon & Montello, 1999; Mattingly, 2005) and wave a magic wand to shift the infrastructure for policing research ethics into a different philosophical frame. Researchers (and the chairs of Research Ethics

Committees) need to get narrative ethics on the table within the existing procedural system. I suggest three rules of thumb, based entirely on personal experience.

1 Tell as many stories as you can. Tell them about yourself, about the research study and about the potential participants. The more you get the ethics committee members thinking within particular stories, the more their judgements will take account of real or potential particularities and specifics. And the less you talk in terms of general principles and rigid protocols, the less you will be judged purely by those principles or held to those protocols. Although many sections of the application forms for research ethics and governance are in tick-box format, there is still plenty of scope for inserting explanations, footnotes and even entire Appendices, all of which may contain stories.

2 Use every opportunity to demonstrate your own research virtues. For example, when asked a question about how you will seek consent from patients, answer with an example (in story form, of course) about how you *did* (in a previous project) demonstrate sensitivity, reflexivity, cultural awareness, and so on. Although you will also be expected to answer the question from a principle-based perspective ('we will seek to respect autonomy', etc.), once the committee members are convinced that you are a virtuous actor in this research story, they will usually start to help you to construct a story that takes your research forward rather than one that cuts it off in its prime. The demonstration of research virtues is best done by someone with plenty of stories up their sleeve, which is why it's never a good idea to send an inexperienced member of the team to field the questions at a Research Ethics Committee review.

3 When submitting example copies of forms and other administrative artefacts, make liberal use of sentences such as 'this form [or whatever] will be adapted as needed by the Chief Investigator to take account of any particular circumstances that emerge during the course of the study'. Your ethics committee may require you to inform them of all such changes that actually occur, but in practice this sort of amendment tends to be undertaken by 'chair's action' – in other words, each ongoing decision will rest in the hands of one individual, whom you must make it your duty to keep informed of the research story as it unfolds. Your original emphasis on the need to respond to the particular can be used to justify the subsequent use of *narrative* judgements by yourself and the chair of the committee.

Having said all that, what is really needed is a programme of research into the very laudable attempt by institutions and professional bodies to make research more 'ethical', and the impact of different theoretical models and practical approaches on the *actual* process and outcome of research. Now there's a radical suggestion with which to end this book!

References

Angelelli C (2005) *Medical Interpreting and Cross-Cultural Communication*. Cambridge: Cambridge University Press.

Aristotle (1996a) *Nicomachean Ethics*. Harmondsworth: Penguin.

Aristotle (1996b) *Poetics* (translated by M Heath). Harmondsworth: Penguin.

Aristotle (2005) *Rhetoric* (translated by H Lawson). Harmondsworth: Penguin.

Atkinson P (1997) Narrative turn or blind alley? *Qual Health Res.* **7**, 325–344.

Atkinson P, Coffey A & Delamont S (2003) *Key Themes in Qualitative Research: continuities and changes*. London: AltaMira.

Baicker K & Chandra A (2004) Medicare spending, the physician workforce, and beneficiaries' quality of care. *Health Affairs*. **7 April**, W4–W196.

Bakhtin M (1984) *Problems of Dostoevsky's Poetics*. Manchester: Manchester University Press.

Balint M (1959) *The Doctor, his Patient and the Illness*. London: Pitman.

Bandura A (1986) *Social Foundations of Thought and Action*. Englewood Cliffs, NJ: Prentice-Hall.

Bandura A (1995) *Self-Efficacy in Changing Societies*. New York: Cambridge University Press.

Bate P (1994) *Strategies for Cultural Change*. Oxford: Butterworth-Heinemann.

Bate P (2000) Synthesizing research and practice: using the action research approach in health care settings. *Soc Policy Admin.* **34**, 478–493.

Bate P (2004) The role of stories and storytelling in organisational change efforts: a field study. In: B Hurwitz, T Greenhalgh & V Skultans (eds) *Narrative Research in Health and Illness*. London: BMJ Publications.

Bate SP, Bevan H & Robert G (2005) *Towards a Million Change Agents: a review of the social movements literature*. London: NHS SDO Programme.

Beauchamp TL & Childress JL (2001) *Principles of Biomedical Ethics* (5e). Oxford: Oxford University Press.

Bligh H (1999) Persistent attenders and heartsink. *Med Educ.* **33**, 398.

Boje DM (1991) The storytelling organization: a study of story performance in an office-supply firm. *Admin Sci Q.* **36**, 106–126.

Boje DM (2001) *Narrative Methods for Organizational and Communication Research*. London: Sage.

Bridger F (2002) *A Charmed Life: the spirituality of Potterworld*. London: Darton Longman & Todd.

Bruner J (1986) *Actual Minds, Possible Words*. Cambridge, MA: Harvard University Press.

Bruner J (1990) *Acts of Meaning*. Cambridge, MA: Harvard University Press.

Buckler SA & Zein C (1996) The spirituality of innovation: learning from stories. *J Product Innovation Manage.* **September**, 391–405.

Burke K (1945) *A Grammar of Motive.* Berkeley, CA: University of California Press.

Bury M, Newbould J & Taylor D (2005) *A Rapid Review of the Current State of Knowledge Regarding Lay-Led Self-Management of Chronic Illness.* London: National Institute for Clinical Excellence.

Byrne PS & Long BEL (1976) *Doctors Talking to Patients.* London: HMSO.

Cavan D & Cradock S (2004) Structured education programmes and type 2 diabetes. *Diabet Med.* **21 (Suppl. 1)**, 10–12.

Chambers I (2005) Applied ethnography. In: NK Denzin & YS Lincoln (eds) *Sage Handbook of Qualitative Research* (3e). London: Sage.

Charon R (2001) Narrative medicine: form, function, and ethics. *Ann Intern Med.* **134**, 83–87.

Charon R (2004) The ethicality of narrative medicine. In: B Hurwitz, T Greenhalgh & V Skultans (eds) *Narrative Research in Health and Illness.* London: BMJ Publications.

Charon R & Montello M (1999) Framing the case: narrative approaches for healthcare ethics committees. *HEC Forum.* **11**, 6–15.

Charon R & Montello M (2002) *Stories Matter: the role of narrative in medical ethics.* London: Routledge.

Cochrane Collaboration (2004) *Cochrane Reviewers' Handbook 4.2.2.* Chichester: John Wiley & Sons Ltd.

Cox K (2001) Stories as case knowledge; case knowledge as stories. *Med Educ.* **35**, 818–819.

Czarniawska B (1998) *A Narrative Approach to Organization Studies.* Qualitative Research Methods Series 43. London: Sage.

Department of Health (2001) *The Expert Patient: a new approach to chronic disease management for the twenty-first century.* London: Department of Health.

Derrida J (1974) *Of Grammatology.* Baltimore, MD: Johns Hopkins University Press.

Elwyn G & Gwyn R (1999) Stories we hear, and stories we tell: analysing talk in clinical practice. *BMJ.* **318**, 186–188.

Elwyn G, Greenhalgh T & Macfarlane F (2000) *Groups: a hands-on guide to small group work in education, management and research.* Oxford: Radcliffe Medical Press.

Elwyn G, Hocking H, Burtonwood A *et al.* (2002) Learning to plan? A critical fiction about the facilitation of professional and practice development plans in general practice. *J Interprofess Care.* **16**, 349–358.

Eraut M (1999) Non-formal learning, implicit learning and tacit knowledge. In: F Coldfield (ed.) *Informal Learning.* Bristol: Policy Press.

Eve R (2003) *PUNs and DENs: discovering learning needs in general practice.* Oxford: Radcliffe Medical Press.

Fontana A & Frey J (2005) From structured questions to negotiated text. In: NK

Denzin & YS Lincoln (eds) *Sage Handbook of Qualitative Research* (3e). London: Sage.

Foucault M (1973) *The Birth of the Clinic: an archaeology of medical practice*. London: Tavistock.

Frank A (1991) *At the Will of the Body: perspectives on illness*. Boston, MA: Houghton Mifflin.

Frank A (1995) *The Wounded Storyteller: body, illness, and ethics*. Chicago: University of Chicago Press.

Frank A (1998) Just listening: narrative and deep illness. *Fam Systems Health.* **16**, 197–216.

Friere P (1974) *Education for Critical Consciousness*. New York: Continuum.

Gabriel Y (2000) *Storytelling in Organisations: facts, fictions and fantasies.* Oxford: Oxford University Press.

Gabriel Y (2004) The voice of experience and the voice of the expert – can they speak to each other? In: B Hurwitz, T Greenhalgh & V Skultans (eds) *Narrative Research in Health and Illness.* London: BMJ Publications.

Gardner H (1995) *Leading Minds: an anatomy of leadership*. London: Harper Collins.

Geertz C (1973) *The Interpretation of Cultures*. New York: Basic Books.

Geertz C (1988) *Works and Lives*. Stanford, CA: Stanford University Press.

General Medical Council (1995) *Duties of a Doctor*. London: British Medical Association.

Goffman E (1969) *The Presentation of Self in Everyday Life*. New York: Penguin.

Goffman E (1981) *Forms of Talk*. Oxford: Blackwell.

Gomm R, Hammersley M & Foster P (2000) *Case Study Method*. London: Sage.

Good B (1994) *Medicine, Rationality and Experience*. New York: Cambridge University Press.

Good M-JDV, Brodwin PE, Good BJ *et al.* (1994) *Pain as Human Experience: an anthropological perspective*. Berkeley, CA: University of California Press.

Greenhalgh T (1999) Narrative-based medicine: narrative-based medicine in an evidence-based world. *BMJ.* **318**, 323–325.

Greenhalgh T (2001) Storytelling should be targeted where it is known to have greatest added value. *Med Educ.* **35**, 818–819.

Greenhalgh T (2002) Intuition and evidence – uneasy bedfellows? *Br J Gen Pract.* **52**, 395–400.

Greenhalgh T & Hurwitz B (1999) Narrative-based medicine: why study narrative? *BMJ.* **318**, 48–50.

Greenhalgh T & Collard A (2003) *Sharing Stories: a new approach to multiprofessional training in diabetes care*. London: BMJ Publishing Group.

Greenhalgh T, Helman C & Chowdhury AM (1998) Health beliefs and folk models of diabetes in British Bangladeshis: a qualitative study. *BMJ.* **316**, 978–983.

Greenhalgh T, Robert G, Macfarlane F *et al.* (2004) Diffusion of innovations in service organisations: systematic literature review and recommendations for future research. *Millbank Q.* **82**, 581–629.

Greenhalgh T, Collard A & Begum N (2005a) Sharing stories: complex intervention for diabetes education in minority ethnic groups who do not speak English. *BMJ*. **330**, 628.

Greenhalgh T, Robert G, Macfarlane F *et al.* (2005b) Storylines of research in diffusion of innovation: a meta-narrative approach to systematic review. *Soc Sci Med.* **61**, 417–430.

Greenhalgh T, Russell J & Swinglehurst D (2005c) Narrative methods in quality improvement research. *Qual Safety Health Care*. **14**, 443–449.

Gubrium JF & Holstein JA (1998) Narrative practice and the coherence of personal stories. *Sociol Q.* **39**, 163–187.

Gwyn R (2002) *Communicating Health and Illness*. London: Sage.

Habermas J (1987) *The Theory of Communicative Action*. Boston, MA: Beacon.

Hamm RM (2003) Medical decision scripts: combining cognitive scripts and judgement strategies to account fully for medical decision making. In: D Hardman & L Macchi (eds) *Thinking: psychological perspectives on reasoning, judgement and decision making*. London: John Wiley & Sons.

Hammersley M (2001) *Some Questions About Evidence-Based Practice in Education*. Leeds: Annual Conference of the British Educational Research Association, University of Leeds.

Handy C (1993) *Understanding Organisations*. London: Penguin.

Heath I (1997) *The Mystery of General Practice*. London: Nuffield Provincial Hospital Trust.

Higgins JM & McAllaster C (2002) Want innovation? Then use cultural artefacts that support it. *Organiz Dynamics*. **31**, 74–84.

Hinchman LP & Hinchman SK (1997) *Memory, Identity, Community: the idea of narrative in the human sciences*. Albany, NY: State University of New York Press.

Holstein JA & Gubrium JF (2000) *The Self We Live By: narrative identity in a postmodern world*. New York: Oxford University Press.

Humphreys JM & Brown AD (2002) Narratives of organisational identity and identification: a case study of hegemony and resistance. *Organiz Studies*. **23**, 421–447.

Hunter KM (1991) *Doctors' Stories: the narrative structure of medical knowledge*. Princeton, NJ: Princeton University Press.

Iedema R, Flabouris A, Grant S *et al.* (2006) Narrativizing errors of care: critical incident reporting in clinical practice. *Soc Sci Med.* **62**, 133–144.

Iles V & Sutherland K (1998) *Organisational Change*. London: NHS SDO Programme.

Jewkes R (2002) Preventing domestic violence. *BMJ*. **324**, 253–254.

Jones AH (1998) Narrative in medical ethics. In: T Greenhalgh & B Hurwitz (eds) *Narrative-Based Medicine: dialogue and discourse in clinical practice*. London: BMJ Publications.

Jones SH (2005) Autoethnography: making the personal political. In: NK Denzin & YS Lincoln (eds) *Sage Handbook of Qualitative Research* (3e). London: Sage.

Kirmayer L (2000) Broken narratives: clinical encounters and the poetics of illness experience. In: C Mattingly & LC Garro (eds) *Narrative and the Cultural Construction of Illness and Healing*. Berkeley, CA: University of California Press.

Kleinmann A (1988) *The Illness Narratives: suffering, healing and the human condition*. New York: Basic Books.

Klevens J & Sadowski L (2005) Domestic violence towards women. *Clin Evidence*. **2**, 2293–2302.

Kling J (1995) *Narratives of possibility: social movements, collective stories, and the dilemmas of practice*. Paper presented to the New Social Movement and Community Organising Conference, University of Washington School of Social Work, Washington, DC.

Koev DJ, Tankova TI & Kozlovski PG (2003) Effect of structured group education on glycemic control and hypoglycemia in insulin-treated patients. *Diabetes Care*. **26**, 251.

Kolb DA (1993) The process of experiential learning. In: M Thorpe, R Edwards & A Hanson (eds) *Culture and Processes of Adult Learning*. London: Routledge.

Kuhn TS (1962) *The Structure of Scientific Revolutions*. Chicago: University of Chicago Press.

Labov W (1982) Speech actions and reactions in personal narrative. In: D Tannen (ed.) *Analyzing Discourse: text and talk*. Washington, DC: Georgetown University Press.

Launer J (2002) *Narrative-Based Primary Care: a practical guide*. Oxford: Radcliffe Medical Press.

McDrury J & Alterio M (2002) *Learning Through Storytelling in Higher Education: using reflection and experience to improve learning*. Auckland: Routledge Falmer.

MacIntyre A (1982) *After Virtue*. London: Gerald Duckworth & Co.

MacLure M (2003) *Discourse in Educational and Social Research*. Buckingham: Open University Press.

MacLure M (2005) 'Clarity bordering on stupidity': where's the quality in systematic review? *J Educ Policy*. **20**, 393–416.

Marinker M (1978) The chameleon, the judas goat and the cuckoo. *J R Coll Gen Pract*. **28**, 199–206.

Marmot MG (2003) Understanding social inequalities in health. *Perspect Biol Med*. **46**, S9–23.

Mattingly C (1998) *Healing Dramas and Clinical Plots: the narrative structure of experience*. New York: Cambridge University Press.

Mattingly C (2005) Towards a vulnerable ethics of research practice. *Health*. **9**, 453–472.

Mattingly C & Garro LC (2000) *Narrative and Cultural Construction of Illness and Healing*. Berkeley, CA: University of California Press.

Mishler EG (1984) *The Discourse of Medicine: dialectics of medical interviews*. Norwood, NJ: Ablex.

Mishler EG (1999) *Storylines: craft artists' narratives of identity.* Cambridge, MA: Harvard University Press.

Morley CJ, Thornton AJ, Cole TJ *et al.* (1991) Symptoms and signs in infants younger than 6 months of age correlated with the severity of their illness. *Pediatrics.* **88**, 1119–1124.

Muller J (1999) Narrative approaches to qualitative research in primary care. In: BF Crabtree & L Miller (eds) *Doing Qualitative Research.* London: Sage.

Murdoch JC (1997) Mackenzie's puzzle – the cornerstone of teaching and research in general practice. *Br J Gen Pract.* **47**, 656–658.

Murray SA, Boyd K, Kendall M *et al.* (2002) Dying of lung cancer or cardiac failure: a community-based, prospective qualitative interview study of patients and their carers. *BMJ.* **325**, 929–932.

Newton AZ (1995) *Narrative Ethics.* London, MA: Harvard University Press.

Nussbaum M (2001) *Upheavals of Thought: the intelligence of emotions.* Cambridge: Cambridge University Press.

Pawson R (2002) Evidence-based policy: the promise of 'realist synthesis'. *Evaluation.* **8**, 340–358.

Pawson R, Greenhalgh T, Harvey G *et al.* (2005) Realist review – a new method of systematic review designed for complex policy interventions. *J Health Serv Res Policy.* **10 (Suppl. 1)**, 21–34.

Penny WJ (2001) Patient delay in calling for help: the weakest link in the chain of survival? *Heart.* **85**, 121–122.

Polanyi M (1962) *The Tacit Dimension.* New York: Anchor Day.

Pope C (2003) Resisting evidence: a study of evidence-based medicine as a contemporary social movement. *Health.* **7**, 267–282.

Ricoeur P (1984) *Time and Narrative. Volume 1.* Chicago: University of Chicago Press.

Riessman CK (1990) Strategic uses of narrative in the presentation of self and illness. *Soc Sci Med.* **30**, 1195–1200.

Riessman CK (2001) Analysis of personal narratives. In: JF Gubrium & JA Holstein (eds) *Handbook of Interview Research.* London: Sage.

Riessman CK (2005) Exposing ethics: a narrative about narrative research in India. *Health.* **9**, 473–490.

Royal Pharmaceutical Society of Great Britain (1997) *From Compliance to Concordance. Achieving shared goals in medicine taking.* London: Royal Pharmaceutical Society of Great Britain.

Rubin SB (2002) Beyond the authoritative voice: casting a wide net in ethics consultation. In: R Charon & M Montello (eds) *Stories Matter: the role of narrative in medical ethics.* London: Routledge.

Salinsky J (2002) *Medicine and Literature: the doctor's companion to the classics.* London: Routledge.

Scambler G (2001) *Habermas, Critical Theory and Health.* London: Routledge.

Schuller T, Preston J, Hammond C *et al.* (2004) *The Benefits of Learning. The impact of education on health, family life and social capital.* London: Routledge Farmer.

Senge P (1994) *The Fifth Discipline: the art and practice of the learning organisation.* New York: Doubleday.

Simons H (1996) The paradox of case study. *Camb J Educ.* **26**, 225–240.

Stake R (1996) *The Art of Case Study Research.* London: Sage.

Stone-Mediatore S (2003) *Reading Across Borders: storytelling and knowledge of resistance.* New York: Palgrave Macmillan.

Thor J, Whitlow K, Herrlin B *et al.* (2004) Learning helpers: how they facilitated improvement and improved facilitation. Lessons from a hospital-wide quality improvement initiative. *Qual Manage Health Care.* **30**, 60–74.

Timmons S (2001) How does professional culture influence the success or failure of IT implementation in health services? In: L Ashburner (ed.) *Organisational Behaviour and Organisational Studies in Health Care: reflections on the future.* Basingstoke: Palgrave.

Towle A & Godolphin W (1999) Framework for teaching and learning informed shared decision making. *BMJ.* **319**, 766–771.

Trento M, Passera P, Bajardi M *et al.* (2002) Lifestyle intervention by group care prevents deterioration of Type II diabetes: a 4-year randomized controlled clinical trial. *Diabetologia.* **45**, 1231–1239.

Turner V (1980) Social dramas and stories about them. *Crit Inquiry.* **7**, 141–168.

Turner V (1986) *The Anthropology of Performance.* Urbana, IL: University of Illinois Press.

Van Maanen J (1988) *Tales of the Field: on writing ethnography.* Chicago: University of Chicago Press.

Warlow C (2005) Over-regulation of clinical research: a threat to public health. *Clin Med.* **5**, 33–38.

Waterman H, Tillen D, Dickson R *et al.* (2001) Action research: a systematic review and guidance for assessment. *Health Technol Assess.* **5**, iii–157.

Webb S (2001) Some considerations on the validity of evidence-based practice in social work. *Br J Soc Work.* **31**, 57–79.

Weber M (1947) *The Theory of Social and Economic Organisations* (translated by AM Henderson & T Parsons). Glencoe: Free Press.

Weick KE (1995) *Sensemaking in Organizations.* Thousand Oaks, CA: Sage.

Wenger E (1996) *Communities of Practice: learning, meaning and identity.* Cambridge: Cambridge University Press.

Whittaker E (2005) Adjudicating entitlements: the emerging discourses of research ethics boards. *Health.* **9**, 513–535.

Winter R & Munn Giddings C (2001) *A Handbook for Action Research in Health and Social Care.* London: Routledge.

Yin RK (1994) *Case Study Research: design and methods* (2e). London: Sage.

Index